Practical Approaches to Dramatherapy

# Practical Approaches to Dramatherapy
## The Shield of Perseus

*Madeline Andersen-Warren
and Roger Grainger*

Preface by Anna Seymour

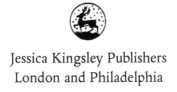

Jessica Kingsley Publishers
London and Philadelphia

The right of Madeline Andersen-Warren and Roger Grainger to be identified as authors of this work has been asserted by them in accordance with the Copyright, Designs and Patents Act 1988.

First published in the United Kingdom in 2000 by
Jessica Kingsley Publishers
116 Pentonville Road
London N1 9JB, UK
and
400 Market Street, Suite 400
Philadelphia, PA 19106, USA

*www.jkp.com*

Copyright © Madeline Andersen-Warren and Roger Grainger 2000
Printed digitally since 2005

**Library of Congress Cataloging in Publication Data**
Grainger, Roger, 1944–
Dramatherapy : expanding horizons / Roger Grainger and Madeline Andersen-Warren.
p.    cm.
Includes bibliographical references and index.
ISBN 1-85302-660-3 (pb. and alk. paper)
1. Psychodrama. I. Andersen-Warren, Madeline, 1948– II. Title.
RC489.P7G692   2000
616.89'1523--dc21                                      99-39963
                                                            CIP

**British Library Cataloguing in Publication Data**
A CIP catalogue record for this book is available from the British Library

ISBN-13: 978 1 85302 660 7
ISBN-10: 1 85302 660 3

# Contents

*Dedicated to Ron English*

Perseus fixed his eyes on Medusa's reflection in his shield. With a single stroke of the Adamantine sickle that Athene had given him, he struck off the Gorgon's head...

(Robert Graves, Greek Myths, 1981, p.69)

I was unable to look directly at the monsters in my life. To confront them would turn me to stone. The fear was paralysing. Yet I needed to conquer them. By using my creativity I could find other ways of approaching the things that frightened me so much.

(A dramatherapy client)

---

With special thanks to Joanne Beals, Vera Byrne, John Casson, Mary Duggan, Doreen Grainger, Terry Haywood, David Henry, Dorothy Iredale, David Kennard, John Rowbottom and Denise Sykes. Extra thanks to Sue Hallam and Kim Dent-Brown for reminding us of the story of the elephant. And also to everyone who has contributed to the author's enthusiasm for dramatherapy.

**Authors' note**

The case studies are inspired by our dramatherapy practice, but are not actual transcripts.

# Preface

What I like about this plain speaking book is that it gets down to the fundamentals of dramatherapy in a clear and unstuffy way, because as it states dramatherapy is about 'participation rather than clinical detachment' (p.218). The authors emphasise how the therapeutic alliance between therapist and client is made through awakening creativity, albeit in the midst of anxiety and distress. Brecht says:

> Mere catastrophe is a bad teacher. One learns hunger and thirst from it, but seldom hunger for truth and thirst for knowledge. No amount of illness will turn a sick man into a physician. (Brecht 1964, p.209)

Yet this is what dramatherapists dare to do, to 'turn the sick man into a physician.'

The theatre is sometimes seen as the pursuit of the bourgeois classes but this book demonstrates how it may be regarded a necessary art in the process of healing available to everyone. There is an essential democracy about the approaches described here that allows space for exploration and development. Dramatherapy as examined in this book does not assume that life can be compared with a play where there is a fixed role for each person, where enactments reinforce the prevailing hierarchy, or where outcomes are inevitable. The ethic of this book sees drama as part of being human, about truth, not deception, and most importantly about choice. It is clear then that, while scripts exist for life and plays are already written, in the dramatherapy space new 'plays' are created wherein endless possibilities for experimentation lie and the outcome is always unknown. As the authors state 'Dramatherapy certainly involves role play, but it is a very different thing from using drama as a way of teaching set patterns of interpersonal behaviour or the correct formulae for what somebody else thinks is the appropriate kind of verbal response within a particular situation' (p.28).

This book encourages dramatherapists to consider their own 'artistry' without sacrificing the crucial relationship with the rigours of the art form. It is most definitely not a 'handbook' in the sense that while it describes practice in detail this is intended to be exemplary rather than proscriptive, conveying 'the expansive spirit of dramatherapy; its fundamental flexibility rather than its availability as a collection of techniques… This flexibility comes from the fact that it is based on a fundamental human principle – the way in which we use imagination to transform and humanise the world we live in' (p.222). So the authors are not simply interested in drama techniques, such as role play, games and 'warm-up' exercises, but in the whole vocabulary of theatrical process, from rehearsal to staging, from genre to the use of theatrical space. The point is that dramatherapists approach the use of theatre with a commitment to change by examining every particular of the context in which they are working to try to find out what is required.

What begins as 'empty space' may be populated by whole worlds of experience, worlds that may not be immediately understood by the dramatherapist, which enable the pain of chaos to emerge and be inhabited within the safe space of dramatic metaphor. Dramatherapists 'have learnt by experience that using imagination in a dramatic way allows us to take our chaos seriously and not turn our backs on it: because the only way to make sense out of our nonsense is to "stay with it"' (p.131).

Or, in Sue Jennings oft quoted phrase, to 'stay with the chaos and the meaning will emerge.' Indeed the authors remind us that in the dramatherapy session is a space uniquely capable of facing chaos, realising that it is a prerequisite for change, that old orders need to go as an 'essential condition for the emergence of new life' (p.123). Thus it is that clients can find acceptance within dramatherapy for their darkest fears and this is amply demonstrated in Madeline Andersen-Warren's description of working with Tourneur's *The Revenger's Tragedy* (Gibbon 1967). This impressive piece of work enables a direct connection to be made between the 'public art' of theatre in the main house at Stratford and the 'making public' of personal distress in the dramatherapy processes 'in contrast to the private fantasy solutions we use to avoid contact with reality in our efforts to hide from life. This is the public use of creative imagination, to join not divide…' (p.222).

The changes that need to be made exist both within and without, and it is important to be reminded that 'we often forget…we have the power to alter…the plot of the whole social drama' (p.56). This book acknowledges both the socio-political context of dramatherapy process and also the fact that its theatrical roots are themselves socially generated. The theatrical forms and structures used are therefore not immutable. The intention is not to use the 'containment' of the drama to seduce, avoid or deceive, but rather to contribute to an ever-expanding horizon of therapeutic possibilities in practice.

Since it is a book about 'approaches', each chapter has a specific focus addressing issues of methodology, content, interpretation and purpose. Its strength lies in the ability of the authors to speak about complex processes with clarity and thereby locate what distinguishes dramatherapy from other forms of therapeutic intervention. In particular the detailed description of one to one work provides unique insight.

In 1994 I was in Moscow to deliver a paper at the World Congress of the International Federation for Theatre Research: I was struck by a colleague's paper, 'Theatre as a Seismograph of Society'. Jon Nygaard's thesis was that we should take seriously what is going on in the theatre because often it is there that stories are told of what is to come, that dramas are played out in the fiction of theatre before taking place in reality. He cited a number of examples that prefigured the eastern European 'revolutions' and in particular the work of Vaclav Havel. It would be wrong to think of the theatre as a place for fortune telling, none the less, I find Nygaard's thesis attractive because it suggests some significant things about the theatre that can often be overlooked and that I would propose are important to the dramatherapist.

The physical shaping and production of drama causes professional theatre makers to ask questions about the 'needs' of audiences. These might be interpreted as perceived or actual needs and the size of box office returns might well play a crucial role in this process. However the popularity of even the crassest musical will tell us something about the world we live in. Trends and influences in the theatre and indeed popular culture will reveal current anxieties and aspirations which become displaced onto cultural 'product'. The client will bring these images, musical themes and ideas into the therapeutic space. Dramatherapy is clear that drama is an essential part of human development and that in most cases, its vocabulary, though it may lie dormant, is potential available for action. Nevertheless, the languages of the public sphere may superimpose this vocabulary. The ways in which public representation of individual experience may either reflect or distort it are important. In the drama-therapy process individuals who feel at odds with the world may struggle with how to express these feelings. In doing so they can be encouraged to relearn the games of stepping into someone else's shoes, telling stories and making imaginary environments, but if they are adults, these metaphorical excursions will also be influenced by a myriad of cultural influences all of which carry with them ideological inferences.

In dramatherapy, we try to discover what are the 'necessary' dramas to be made. What are the 'plays' that need to be 'written' which will enable the client to move forward? In this process there will be countless revolutions, as 'old orders' are swept away to make space for the new, where individuals realise that they can empower themselves to make choices in relation to others. This social dimension of drama exists even in one to one work and the framing provided by dramatic structure, whether in public spaces or the confidentiality of the dramatherapy process, provides a means of ascribing value and form to the chaos of life.

This book provides a consistent, thorough guide to practice, and therefore a basis for others to grow from, in developing the field of work. It may inspire practising and future dramatherapists with the astonishing breadth of dramatherapy in its intellectual and practical challenges.

In the new century, isolation and loneliness are dominant themes, we face profound unease. Dramatherapy has an important role to play with its unique ability to encompass both the private and the social. 'To discover what hurts us so much, the very thing that cuts us off from other people and makes us feel different, rejected, inferior, hopeless is in fact the pledge of our belonging…[it] dignifies our suffering in a way that nothing else can' (p.148). The Dramatherapist needs to be both humble and audacious, an artist, explorer and seeker of social justice. The authors of this book share these qualities and aspirations in abundance and I am proud to name myself as a colleague and friend to both.

*Anna Seymour*
*Manchester June 2000*

# Preface

There is a well-known story about some people who had to say what an elephant was. Unfortunately they were all wearing blindfolds, so they could not see it *was* an elephant. The first one ran up against one of its legs: 'It's a tree,' he said. The second stretched out his hands and felt along its body: 'No, it's not. It's a wall,' she said. Number three felt its ear flapping against her face: 'This is a windmill,' she said. 'No, it's definitely a snake,' said the man who was feeling the trunk. And so on. They never really saw the actual elephant because they were all hung up on its various parts.

We think dramatherapy is like this. If we stand back and look at the whole, we see something which is made up of a lot of different strands but in itself makes up a very recognisable unity. The unity of dramatherapy lies in drama-theatre. When we speak about theatre we are using a word which encompasses a whole range of activities – from the Vienna Opera to glove puppets, from ancient Greek tragedy to French farce. When we speak about drama we mean a form of communication which all human beings use in all sorts of ways, all the time – something very fundamental indeed.

In this book we have set out to illustrate some of the essential strands which make up dramatherapy while preserving its unity as a form of dramatic creativity. This particular elephant is a talented animal, capable of imagination and sensitivity, and exceptionally good at adapting its skills to the needs of particular situations concerning people. In terms of this book, this means that none of the exercises or processes described is to be transferred from the page to the situation of an actual client group or an individual client without carefully adapting it to meet the special needs of the people concerned. We have imagined different ways in which the dramatherapy approach can come into its own, but all situations involving people are different, all are unique, so you will always have to find your own way of making sure that what we describe here will speak to the individuals and groups you are trying to help. This is not a handbook so much as an ideas book. In order to use it properly, the way it is intended to be used, you will need ideas of your own. You will have to think carefully about how you yourself intend to use it. Drama is a powerful medium, even when it seems to be quite ordinary and domestic. In fact, that is when it can be most powerful. You may find this elephant a marvellous friend, but you will never succeed in wholly domesticating it.

# Introduction

Traditions of healing through drama are at least as old as civilisation. Indeed, they appear to be as old as community itself. Because they are non-medical, operating principally through the human understanding, they are to be seen within the context of a philosophy of life, a corporate philosophy inspiring a corporate event. In classical and pre-classical times, dramatic healing was explicitly associated with religion, and this has been so from time to time in succeeding ages. It has taken many forms, from the Greek cult of Esklepius at Epidaurus, and other theatre-based cathartic approaches such as those practised in India and Japan, to the healing shrines of Eleusis, Delphi and Lourdes. In fact, it is as old as the Shamanistic techniques still practised in Tibet and South East Asia (Nilsson 1964; Scheff 1979).

It seems, however, that there is no fundamental reason why its underlying philosophy has to be explicitly religious. The most celebrated explanation of the therapeutic effect of drama — Aristotle's theory of catharsis — does not mention divine personages or influences. What it depends on is human fellow-feeling. Fear for oneself and pity for another person or people are transformed into positive, healing emotions by the experience of encounter that drama contrives. It is as if the circumstances of the drama intensify our natural ability to put ourselves into somebody else's place by demonstrating to us that it is precisely our separateness that allows us to do so. There is a good deal of literature on the subject of catharsis. Critics have wanted to know, for example, how we could possibly be 'purged' (Aristotle's phrase) *of* our feelings *by* our feelings (Lucas 1946). The aim of psychotherapy, however, is to allow hidden emotions to attain full awareness. Drama helps us to share the things that disturb our peace, things that we would rather not face, and to do so in safety. S.H. Butcher (1951), writing in the mid-twentieth century, describes the process as follows: 'The emotion of fear is profoundly altered when it is transformed from the real to the imaginative world. It is no longer the direct apprehension of misfortune hanging over our own life – it is the sympathetic shudder we feel for those whose character in essentials resembles our own' (Butcher 1951, p.258).

In other words, dramatic catharsis depends upon aesthetic distance: 'The play as theatre production originates in the elemental impulse to leap through transformation over the abyss between I and Thou' (Buber 1957, p.64). Aesthetic distance is the awareness that art is only art, encouraging us to draw nearer to its subject matter of people, events and ideas, all of which are part of our own reality. It provides a safe place for meeting and sharing. At the same time, however, it leads us into a more emotionally satisfying world than ours, one of completeness and balance – the world of the timeless moment that refreshes and reconciles, in which existence gives way to being. Aesthetic distance, the structure of the dramatic event, is responsible for both identification and universalisation, idealising the first while humanising the second. As Wilshire says: 'To stage a drama is to intervene in the circuit of life and to build a model of it which disturbs life even as we find it conforming to the model' (Wilshire 1982, p.209).

The re-emergence of drama as therapy in western culture began in Europe in the nineteenth century with the publication of numerous articles about the healing effect of catharsis, and the building of theatres in psychiatric hospitals in France and Germany. In Russia the dramatic approach associated with Stanislavski was elaborated into 'therapeutic theatre', founded upon the experience of catharsis but involving improvisation and play. The connection between spontaneity and catharsis underlies psychodrama, in which the roles of actor and audience are exchanged over and over again (Moreno's 'role-reversal' technique). Psychodrama is now recognised as an important form of group therapy.

If drama is an expression of human imagination, of the delight we have in playing games with our own and others' reality, it is nevertheless reality-changing in its effect. Explanations of the way that it works suggest a lessening of emotional pressure or a resolution of psychological conflict, through the experience of personal relationship and an enhanced sense of engagement with life, a kind of metaphysical security. These things are true of all forms of drama, not only specially contrived experiments or techniques of 'therapeutic drama'. Without an imaginative frame there can be no drama – and where the frame exists, imagination finds a place of healing (Elam 1988; Goffman 1986).

We tend to associate catharsis with tragedy. It also takes place in comedy and romance, even in satire and farce. There are many permutations of relationship among character, actor and audience, all contrived in distance terms. Where it is least likely it may be most powerful. The theatre of Chekhov is very different from that of Brecht; both stand in contrast to the Japanese Noh plays. The manipulation of various different kinds of reality is their relational skill, contributing to the shock of recognition where it occurs. This is what Buber (1957) means by 'leaping through transformation'. Where naturalism soothes us peacefully into identification, drama that is more self-conscious demands a higher degree of imaginative investment, with a correspondingly higher reward.

Dramatherapy means the therapy that is in drama itself – all drama – and not merely the use of some aspects of drama as therapeutic tools. This is its uniqueness. It is not simply role-reversal, effective though this may be, or social skills training by means of practice in role-play. From this point of view there are important differences between dramatherapy and psychodrama, the most important one being that the latter presents its material as straightforward autobiography, whereas the former tends to be more circumspect in its approach to the real lives of those taking part. Psychodrama's 'plots' are actually true in all their dramatic detail. They aim to present a realistic picture of the protagonists' actual experience of the relationships which most closely and intimately affect them (Blatner 1997). Dramatherapy's characteristic approach, however, is to leave the crucial business of focusing on individual lives to the persons most intimately concerned. The processes described in this book are all ways in which individuals are encouraged to discover their own truths from their own angles. Dramatherapy deliberately chooses to approach these things circumspectly, setting the scene for personal healing without prescribing the treatment for it. It prefers fictional stories to straightforward auto-biography, allowing those taking part to 'sit more easily' to what is unfolding around them, choosing whether or not they want to take it personally by becoming involved to the extent of identifying with the men, women and children, animals, gods and mythical creatures who inhabit the imaginary world created by the group.

The power of dramatic identification makes this a potentially trans-forming experience. For the time that the play lasts we are presented with the opportunity to regard ourselves in a different way as different people, and to do so with an emotional intensity which renders the episode an authentic part of our ongoing experience, able to affect the way in which we will live life in the future. It does not have to do this, of course. We can choose whether or not we allow ourselves to become involved in this way. It is, after all, only a play, and does not pretend to be anything else. Dramatherapy, like theatre, goes out of its way to make the fact quite clear: if we want to lose ourselves in its world we are very welcome to do so. But it is up to us to decide whether and to what degree we are willing to co-operate. Dramatherapy aims to make the choice as safe as possible for us. It does this in the same way that theatre does it – by underlining its own identity as fiction.

Drama, whether it takes place in theatres, dramatherapy sessions or simply in the reader's imagination, depends on being self-proclaimed fiction. Its relevance to ourselves is not immediately obvious. It is a play written to be performed, *being* performed. Dramatherapy works on the principle that this is its greatest therapeutic asset. Drama's meaning is not obvious on purpose. This means that we have to come forward ourselves in the attempt to understand it. In other words, we have to work at it in order to see it from the inside. It is hiding from us as a story about someone else; and this encourages us to come a little closer, explore a little more deeply. In the kind of drama we frequently encounter in dramatherapy, where the fictional characters stand in for entire realms of human experience, not only is the story different from ordinary life – on the surface that is – but also the people in it may seem exotic and bizarre, personages belonging to an entirely different order of being from our own. You may find yourself in a world of heroes and heroines, demons and monsters, goddesses and gods. The refusal of drama to be explicit about its personal relevance to my own experience – its determination to be talking about someone else – has the effect of inducing me to relax my vigilance with regard to things I am willing to think and feel about myself.

At the same time, drama's honesty about its fictional nature and its willingness to be seen as a play defend it against the charge of being a trick, a way of getting under people's guard without asking permission to do so. Drama always asks permission: in some way or other it always manages to get across to us the crucial fact that it is 'only a play'. This is something we must know if we are to be willing to suspend our disbelief.[1] We have to feel safe before we can permit ourselves to run this kind of risk. Dramatherapy is a way of encouraging vulnerable people to look more courageously at the challenges and rewards of becoming more involved with life.

When it comes down to it, dramatherapy's credentials lie in the fact that drama itself is a fundamental human experience. Augusto Boal (1992) describes it as the capacity possessed by human beings to observe themselves in action. This fundamental fact about drama itself means that the scope possessed by dramatherapy as a treatment modality is potentially unlimited. Before we can be healed, we must be able to look at ourselves. In some way or other, we have to be in a position to see ourselves in action as human beings. To be human is not simply to be an organism, a mind and body obviously interconnected, holistically united, but functioning on its own in a relational vacuum. Real individuals are philosophical abstractions. They belong to a way of looking at life which claims to be 'scientific' but turns out in the long run to be considerably less dependable than the telling of stories about the way people relate to and live with one another. We learn about human reality by observing other people and ourselves in action, making sense of what we see in terms of what we ourselves are experiencing. Thus we see life in terms of our own involvement in it, learning the truth about living in the action of reaching across to others, inspired and guided by what we see in them that reminds us of ourselves.

If the meaning and significance of drama is as all-inclusive as that, it follows that dramatherapy itself will be wide-ranging in its relevance. In this book we have set out to do two things. First, we look at the ways in which dramatherapy functions, its credentials as a treatment modality concerned with the healing of persons. We have tried to do this as straightforwardly as possible, beginning with a chapter about the significance of shape in dramatherapy, the reason why things take place in a particular order, and going on to demonstrate how this pattern is used in a variety of ways, all of which are practical and task-applied. Chapter 3 begins a series of chapters which concern the therapeutic action of drama as this is experienced in dramatherapy, and the ways in which a dramatherapy session or course of sessions focuses the healing power of theatre. As a form of therapy, dramatherapy is concerned with human experience of pain and disruption. Consequently, the heart of this part of the book lies in Chapter 5, about chaos, and in Chapter 6, in which we consider the balance between safety and danger which brings a degree of order to chaos and is the locus of cathartic healing. We then go on to look at the actual content of dramatherapy, as meaning, story and text, finishing with Chapter 9 which is devoted to assessment and evaluation – always an important subject when we are dealing with the arts therapies.

The second objective is equally important. This book draws special attention to the flexibility of this approach by describing a range of approaches to group and individual work. There are many books about what dramatherapy is and how it works. This is an essentially practical, hands-on book. For example, social skills training is a recognised category of task-orientated therapeutic intervention; the dramatherapeutic approach works towards the same aims for the client, but in a very different way – a specifically *dramatherapy* way. This is true of many other similar situations illustrated in practical ways throughout the text. The approaches described here are all recognisably dramatherapy approaches even though they are concerned with very different situations and problems.

## Note

1   The phrase 'willing suspension of disbelief' was coined by Coleridge in 1817 (1991, Chapter 14, passion). It is an idea of the very greatest significance for drama and dramatherapy.

# CHAPTER I

# From Safety to Safety

## The Shape of the Dramatherapy Session

Dramatherapy is usually thought of as a special kind of group therapy. Even when, as often happens, a dramatherapy approach is adopted in one-to-one situations, the group therapy idea persists. There is every reason why it should do so. Dramatherapy is always a group phenomenon in the same way, and for the same reasons, that drama itself is essentially a group event, even when only two people are actually present. Although human beings possess the ability to 'act out' dramas in their own imagination and these private scenarios can have any number of characters, actual interpersonal, rather than intra-personal, drama requires at least two people so that there may be a dialogue between them, and each can be aware of the effect his or her presence, and what he or she is doing or saying, has on the other person and vice versa; in other words, so that personal interaction can take place. The fact that every human meeting is a kind of drama, even if it involves only two people, has been noted by social psychologists such as Erving Goffman (1986, 1990).

In his book *The Presentation of Self in Everyday Life* Goffman (1990) draws attention to the 'staged' nature of so many of our social contacts. Not only are our encounters with other people 'little dramas', but also they are actually things that we 'present' one another with in ways that we have no difficulty in recognising once the fact has been drawn to our attention. This element of presentation is in fact vital for all kinds of human dramas, even those that take place in our imagination and are never actually seen by anyone else at all. Those who compare drama with theatre on the grounds that the second involves an audience while the first does not are overlooking this vital fact about being human – that we are creatures who love to present ourselves, in one way or another, and in order to do so we have to find an audience of some kind. Theatre itself is the clearest and most obvious way in which we do this; but we are doing it all the time and will go on doing it until we die. Human awareness is not simply a matter of playing roles in inter- and intra-personal dramas, but of constructing our own personal theatres, theatre being most accurately described as the human ability to look at oneself, acting in the real world. The first organised theatres in western Europe, those of classical Greece, developed out of a cast of two actors – plus an audience.

All this is a way of explaining why it is that dramatherapy is always group therapy, even when it is carried out one-to-one. Like other kinds of dramatically conceived processes, it conjures up its own audience. Not only this, but also it is capable of inventing other members of the cast who are able, although invisible and inaudible, to take on roles as extra members of the group. Drama of any kind is a group happening, binding the people involved in it together in a network of action and reaction which makes up a dramatic event. You could say that drama is itself an action of binding events and people together into some kind of significant happening. It takes various components of social experience, various things happening to people, and focuses our attention on the way they are connected together by the human impulse to make sense of life. By involving people in a specially contrived 'world of the play' in which this kind of connection has been made particularly clear, having been carefully plotted beforehand, drama connects them more closely to ordinary life while appearing to set them apart from it. To construct any kind of drama is to isolate a part of life and then to make it as lifelike as possible by exaggerating and developing the things about it that give life meaning. Actors and audience are united in a living experience of the imagination as they find themselves sharing the things that they hold in common as human beings. In other words, acting as a group.

Another way in which plays create groups has to do with their shape. This follows on from what was said above about 'sectioning off' part of life and giving it a kind of separate existence, to be used as a workshop for human relationship. In order to do this you have to interrupt the ordinary flow of interconnected events and create a kind of special event, something that can be focused on more or less by itself so that what is going on in this place, between these people, in these circumstances, will be immediately apparent – at least at the emotional level, if not always at the intellectual one. We recognise things as events, and are able to concentrate on them without being distracted by whatever may be going on elsewhere, by the space they take up in the flow of time. Timewise, for an event to have shape, it must have three things: a beginning, a middle and an end. In order for us to concentrate our attention properly it must begin and end somewhere, so that it stands out from all the other things that have happened and are going on happening. This may seem rather obvious but it is something that is often overlooked, and in fact it is very important indeed. Plays interrupt life in order to say something about it in its own language. Most ways of commenting on the way people behave and the way things turn out are conclusions drawn about events and solutions; drama on the other hand is always an example of the thing itself – an imaginative reproduction using the authentic materials: human body, mind and spirit seen in action, not merely thought or spoken about. So the space it makes for itself is space *hewn out of life*.

Plays stand by themselves, apart from life. However, they do this by staying part of life, not in theory but in fact. Because the things they depict are real – real feelings, thoughts, ways of acting and reacting – they have their own kind of realism, and we talk about this being 'true to life'; but their realism is not to be confused with ordinary everyday time-bound reality. Any kind of drama stands out as a special event. In order to qualify as an actual piece of drama it must signal its 'special event-ness', just as singers bow before starting to sing and, when they have finished, bow again. In other words drama, in order to be recognised as drama, needs to have a beginning, a middle and an end. When we think about plays we have read or seen or actually taken part in, we remember them as complete in themselves. That is why we remember them. It was about *this*, we say, or about *that*, meaning not that it was vaguely concerned with these things but that it stands out in our memories as being memorable statements concerning them, *actual examples of them*. Drama can have all sorts of implications for us, stir up all kinds of memories, give rise to feelings much deeper and more powerful than those it is actually expressing; but the depth and power of its effect comes from its ability to say something definite and say it concisely, to be a recognisable event not simply part of something else. Plays are focused human experience. Slices of life, in fact.

All this is of great importance for dramatherapists. The impact of drama depends on this focused effect. If dramatherapy is to be genuinely dramatic – to heal by being dramatic – it must not only embody its imaginative content and subject matter, but also reproduce its shape. This needs to be said right at the beginning of a book like this one, which is concerned with the usefulness and practicability of dramatherapy as a treatment modality. Dramatherapy is not simply a way of approaching human problems and difficulties by 'acting them out'. Many kinds of therapies involve using the imagination to conjure up alternative situations and settings to the one being dealt with. Psychotherapists often go out of their way to create a special kind of protected environment in which clients will feel safe and unthreatened by whatever may be going on outside the charmed circle of the therapeutic relationship; having done so, they may well go on to encourage their client to use her or his imagination to recreate events and presences by calling on people present to take on roles which would not normally be theirs, and generally behaving 'as if' (Duggan and Grainger 1997). Psychodrama itself is the most obvious and striking example, of course. So what is different about dramatherapy?

The main difference lies in its shape. Dramatherapy concentrates, deliberately and specifically, on reproducing the shape of drama. It is always drama-shaped, even when its content may not actually be itself very dramatic. In this it closely resembles theatre, which established its identity as make-believe in the clearest and most unmistakable ways. Certainly dramatherapy does not take place in a special kind of building, arranged so as to assert an unmistakable distinction between actors and audience, nor does it necessarily involve things like curtains, screens, stage lights or make-up. Dramatherapy registers the crucial difference between life and art, ordinary experience and the world created by imagination, in ways that are less tangible. All the same, it certainly registers this difference quite systematically and with the same effect on people's experience, and it does so by sticking to the fundamental theatrical process, the thing which characterises all kinds of theatre – the experience of going into something, being in it, and coming out of it, in which the vividness of whatever it is that happens to us in mid-process is governed by and actually depends upon the degree to which we are made conscious of entering into and emerging from it. Theatre is a special time and place, one which we look forward *to* and back *on.* It takes hold of the specialness of drama, its identity as an event on its own, and presents it to the very best advantage, so that it can make its own unique kind of point. Drama and theatre are both essentially things that happen in three stages. They use the power that is implicit in threeness, what Euclid referred to as the 'shape of perfection', having a beginning, a middle and an end.

This is the kind of presentation that dramatherapy uses to give dramatic shape to its subject matter and to draw our attention to things which are usually taken for granted, actions and events and relationships which are caught up in the daily business of what T.S. Eliot (1955, p.10) calls 'living and partly living', moving out of reach before we can bring them into focus. 'What I tell you three times is true,' says the Bellman in Lewis Carroll's *The Hunting of the Snark* (1980, p.1); there is definitely something about the threefold nature of the dramatherapy process that gives it the impact of genuine drama.

A dramatherapy session falls into three parts. This is not an arbitrary division: each part moves into the next. From one point of view it is a continuous process; from another it is a grouping together of three quite different kinds of experiences, each of them more or less distinct from the other two. Thus *Stage 1* consists of preparation for personal involvement with other people, mutual self-disclosure, imaginative adventure along with others into ways of doing, thinking and feeling that may be unfamiliar and consequently a bit alarming because of this. This first stage is characterised by the gradual development of feelings of being able to support and be supported by other members of the group. It corresponds in contracted form to the rehearsal period in theatre or to the moments of preparation that precede actually going on stage. *Stage 2* is more consciously dramatic: scenarios are invented, old situations explored in new ways, roles assumed and abandoned within an experimental framework. Even when the action is not overtly dramatic, people are encouraged to look at the world and the experience of being alive in it in a variety of ways, some of them designed to bring out a sense of wonder at things normally disregarded or taken for granted. The sense of really looking at things, really feeling them, which drama can give, is conjured up by using imagination to present the familiar in unfamiliar ways so that the experience of being alive can regain its impact. In *Stage 3* we return to more ordinary ways of looking at, and being in, the world. If what has gone before, in Stage 2, has involved the exchange of roles among group members or the assumption of fictional identities based on mythical personages of one kind or another, involving a radical shift from everyday reality into an alternative, imaginary, state of affairs, this last part of the dramatherapy process will involve a process of de-roling, during which group members confirm one another in their ordinary identities. This part of a dramatherapy session moves away from the strict theatrical model, as there is no formal de-roling among actors, either professional or amateur. The fall of the curtain, the ceremony of 'taking one's call', is followed by the unceremonious removal of make-up and re-entry into the world waiting beyond the stage door.

This threefold shape is implicit in dramatherapy. Sometimes it becomes explicit, as groups are encouraged to regard an entire session, or course of sessions, as a journey:

1  *Departure*: in which the ultimate destination is agreed upon, and the people involved prepare to embark on it in one another's company.

2  *Voyage*: in which security is exchanged for adventure and everything is in a state of flux between 'here' and 'there', 'now' and 'then'.

3  *Arrival*: in which newness and discovery, the way of experiencing things that has emerged from the symbolic transition of the voyage, is celebrated by those present as a way of embodying the experience of personal change which has taken place during the voyage.

It is not claimed that everybody who takes part in this kind of symbolic 'voyage to higher ground' is automatically transformed by the experience. There is nothing magical about dramatherapy; people are not immediately rendered fully able to cope with themselves and other people by its action. What we are saying here is that this kind of corporate journey of the imagination constitutes a genuine human experience, something lived through and not simply thought about, with the ability to affect future thoughts and attitudes to life. Dramatherapy is always active as an effective symbol of personal change, effective because it is specially designed to be a real event in the lives of those taking part. Its dramatic shape carries with it the immediacy of a specially focused happening in which life is experienced with particular vividness and the experience of an altered way of being oneself comes across as a practical possibility – practical because it has actually happened. Change is something which I have known; at that time, in that place, among these people, I felt it to be a part of my life. Shared imagination carries with it its own reality, its own ability to stay in our minds with all the vividness of personal experience. Some of the most powerful and unforgettable examples of this take place within an artistic setting, particularly one that involves drama.

Because dramatherapy is rooted in artistic experience it always works via the imagination – so that even when it does not involve a corporate drama or piece of group theatre it works hard to create the circumstances in which people taking part can work as creatively as possible with the materials available to them within the resources of a particular group. Always, in dramatherapy, the accent is on discovering ways of looking at life that confirms our awareness of ourselves as playing a part in whatever it is that happens to us, rather than simply being victims of things beyond our control. To regard life in this imaginative way is in fact to treat it as drama – and by doing this we are conscious of exercising a degree of control over it. In drama we call on the power of 'as if' in a way that is purposeful, focused and effective, using shared imagination to affirm our personal reality by giving it the shape necessary to contain change without being destroyed by it.

In the dramatherapy process that follows, shape is the principal theme.

# CHAPTER 2

# Changing Social Behaviour
## Task-Applied Dramatherapy

This book covers a range of ways in which dramatherapy can be used. Indeed its main aim, the purpose of writing it, was to demonstrate how flexible the dramatherapy approach is, and how it can be applied to all kinds of personal and social problems. This chapter concentrates on a particular example of what might be called task-applied dramatherapy, by which is meant the use of dramatherapy in situations in which the problems to be tackled are more or less clearly defined, whether they are regarded as behavioural or cognitive, personal or social. Very probably they are all these things, of course; but the situation as it presents itself seems to call for intervention of a particular kind, designed to bring about a very specific kind of change in the way somebody thinks, feels and behaves – particularly the way they are behaving *now*, which may very well be the cause of the immediate problem.

Just as some questions require immediate answers, some clinical situations call for direct action, undertaken to modify the ways in which individuals (and sometimes whole groups of people) habitually respond to things within the immediate environment which alarm, threaten or disturb them, or are likely to do so in the near future. The ways in which they set about coping with whatever it may be that is so very disturbing may actually have the effect of making things worse, not better; so that if the situation is to be improved at all it is the ways of coping themselves that have to be changed. Clinical psychology has come up with various techniques for this kind of 'behaviour modification'. These range from ways of changing the behaviour itself by altering the stimulus–response linkage, which involves the systematic reinforcement of alternative behavioural responses leaving 'unadaptive' behaviour to 'decay' through lack of reward ('negative reinforcement'), to ways of helping individuals adjust their customary expectations about the kinds of thing that are likely to happen, *the world as they see it being the place it is.* This kind of approach, often associated with personal construct psychology, concentrates on the way we think about life, the study of things we expect to happen, the mental associations we make that govern our assumptions and reactions to other people and ourselves.

In between these two positions, but nearer to the behaviour-modification model, there are various techniques and theories of de-sensitisation which concentrate on the fact that life situations that produce a knee-jerk reaction of recoil, so that we lose our ability to behave in a calm, sometimes even a rational, way and cause ourselves and other people distress by our unsociable behaviour, can be dealt with by depriving these things of their ability to shock and disorientate us. Whether they are insects or animals, places, people or social occasions, actually experiencing them has the effect of reducing their power over us. There are two main ways of putting this idea into action. One is called 'flooding' – the person is plunged right into the middle of whatever it is that appals and terrifies them and so 'learns the hard way' that they are able to survive it *even at its worst.* The other method is much gentler and consists of introducing the person to the loathed presence by a process of carefully graded steps, beginning perhaps with simply talking about it, then looking at pictures, handling something closely associated with it – a hair, perhaps, or a realistic model or, in the case of social phobias, a carefully set up construction of a social scene – until the person is used not only to the idea but also to the actual presence of whatever it was that used to throw them into such inner turmoil and outward panic and confusion. The cognitive-behavioural model of clinical psychology concentrates very much on trying to change our behaviour by affecting our ideas and the way we are accustomed to thinking about things. It is not that we are encouraged to work things out differently (as in personal construct psychology); simply that the experience of getting used to whatever it may be that disturbs us makes us less frightened of it, which is in itself a rewarding experience, setting up a self-reinforcement link which has a knock-on effect upon the way we behave.

In short, all sorts of things exist within the clinical practice of bringing about personal and social change. At first sight the dramatherapy approach to personal and social adjustment seems similar to the cognitive-behavioural one, or the one used by some kinds of occupational therapy, both of which make considerable use of role-play and enactment to model socially acceptable ways of behaving in public. Simulation, modelling and role-play are all widely used therapeutic tools and the attempt to construct an alternative 'social frame' for personal reality has been described as being basic to psychotherapy itself. As Flowers (1975, p.159) puts it, 'The major difficulty in writing about simulation and role playing in psychotherapy and related helping endeavours is that almost all therapy can be viewed as a simulation of the client's real life.' Certainly behavioural psychologists have been using drama as a kind of visual aid for teaching strategies of social interaction for many years now, and mainstream clinical psychology sees enactment as a useful tool for shaping these stimulus–response connections regarded as 'adaptive' for socially acceptable behaviour – and consequently, private peace of mind. Surely this is what dramatherapy aims to do! So what makes it so different?

The difference lies in the way we define drama. Drama and role-play are similar but certainly not identical. Dorothy Langley (1983) sums up the difference when she says that therapeutic drama 'is not an acquired skill which people can or cannot do, but a medium in which each person can participate at his own level'; she goes on to say that dramatherapy is 'an extension of the natural play that we all know as children that gives people the means to become more creative and spontaneous beings' (Langley 1983, p.14). Dramatherapy certainly involves role-play, but it is a very different thing from using drama as a way of teaching set patterns of interpersonal behaviour or the correct formulae for what somebody else thinks is the appropriate kind of verbal response within a particular situation. Task-applied dramatherapy uses our ability to assume roles while holding back from teaching us exactly what roles to adopt. This is because it concentrates upon the kind of dramatic games that, as Erikson (1965) says, are our primary, most fundamental ways of learning how to be human. From being small children, we are used to playing dramatic games with ourselves and other people so that we can discover the ways of behaving *and of being* that suit us best within the 'given circumstances' in which we find ourselves. According to Goffman (1990), we act through various ways of behaving towards ourselves and one another; it is as if we are 'trying life out for size'. It is in this as-if sense that dramatherapy is dramatic. Just as a play is a 'game for the imagination' in which we can choose how much we want to 'be' the characters in the story, so a dramatherapy session leaves us free to learn about ourselves and those around us in our own natural way – which turns out to be a drama-orientated one. Its approach is indirect, via the game, and the task of the therapist is to 'set the scene' without coercing or manipulating those taking part. Therapists aim, with the help and co-operation of their clients, to create a setting in which those present will be able to experience the way they feel, think about and act towards other people and themselves, *and the way they would like to*. If they are going to find the courage to do this they certainly need to feel psychologically safe, safer than they usually feel; a good deal of effort goes into bringing this about, as we saw when we were looking at the shape of dramatherapy sessions in Chapter 1.

According to Blatner and Blatner (1988), the 'special category of playfulness' allows things to be 'real and unreal at the same time', so that the mind 'seems to experience a kind of pleasure in being able to encompass these seemingly irreconcilable opposites' (1988, p.29). Some-how games manage to let us enjoy other people's presence without being frightened or put off by it. It is only a game, so we can play at being friends and reap the benefit of real personal contact. We shall return to this trade-off between safety and danger in later chapters; but now we consider its value in games. One client gave the following reasons for liking to start a session with a group game:

- In a game you have to set some space aside at the beginning of a session to allow yourselves to get to know one another better. It is not like being in a doctor–patient relationship or a pupil–teacher one. It is a special kind of set-up.

- You have to have rules, but this is to make it fair. Besides, they are not like the rules you have in life; they refer only to the game itself. (Rules in real life take you back to being a child, when people had some sort of hold over you and used it.)

- It does not matter if you get mixed up and make mistakes.

- Silly games are the best. Hard games make you think too hard, and they get too competitive.

- The game is for all of is. It is between us. You play it your way, I play it mine, but it is the same game.

- People show what they are really like in a game. You get to know them best in games; you see how they work things out, for instance.

Thus, task-applied dramatherapy does not function by directly imitating a familiar social situation, as in conventional role-play techniques, but by exploring ways of giving people a chance to be more aware of their real relationships with themselves and other people. The dramatherapy approach to problem-solving aims to produce as 'un-clinical' an atmosphere as possible. It tries not to 'do things' to people or allow them to feel like patients, or – worse still – experimental subjects. In this chapter we give an example of a particular kind of task-applied dramatherapy, a series of sessions aimed at helping people to be more assertive in their relationships with others. The activities and discussions described here are geared to this specific end; but the same approach can be used for other 'tasks' apart from 'assertiveness training'. Whatever the main instrumental purpose may be, however, the dramatherapy method always remains the same – one of participation rather than clinical detachment.

People taking part in a dramatherapy session are encouraged to concentrate as hard as they can on what it is that is going on within the group. This applies to everyone involved, group members as well as therapists. As in other kinds of group therapy, this kind of 'detached involvement' (or 'involved detachment') is the main therapeutic method. In dramatherapy, however, a good deal of this conscious attention is devoted to the task of building up the right kind of atmosphere within the group. This is a shared responsibility, in which everybody present, not only the therapist or group leader, must take part. Certainly the initiative comes from the leader, but the kind of activity she or he is likely to suggest will be one in which everyone present plays a part in building group cohesion, so that things begin to go with a swing and people feel at home in whatever it is that is happening. In some cases this may be identifiable as an actual group game, but whatever form it takes, it should always *feel like* a game to those taking part in it, and they are encouraged to enjoy it and relax into playing it.

At the same time, however, they are also encouraged by the therapist to think about what is going on, in themselves and in the group – to try to be objective about their subjective experiences, and to share their ideas and feelings in the same way that they have been sharing the activity they have been involved in. In the exercises which follow, times of group activity alternate with opportunities for discussion and mutual feedback – 'What did it feel like?' and, just as important, 'What did you think it was for?'

In this way, the exchange of ideas and feelings taking place within a context of shared enjoyment and interest builds up an atmosphere of belonging together and having things in common. This may take some effort, particularly with a group of people who may feel very different from one another (and may, of course, actually *be* very different; patients in a psychiatric hospital, for instance, represent a range of socio-economic groupings, ages, clinical diagnoses and personality types, apart from considerations such as 'how things are going this morning' and 'who you remind me of', which are entirely unpredictable and can be crucial). The function of the game turns out to be vitally important for the entire dramatherapy process because it is able to override some of these factors and create a mini-culture of trust and acceptance on which depends people's willingness, and even their ability to revise their attitude towards the possibility of change. This 'safe place' is only a temporary structure, of course, but it is one that can be revisited from time to time so that its significance as an important personal experience grows, and the fact that it is a special kind of happening, not the sort of thing you get involved with every day, can make it even more vivid. These experiences are transitory but powerful, and they can have a lasting effect on people's attitudes towards and feelings about themselves, other people and life in general.

Some of the changes in experience and behaviour reported by those who have taken part in this kind of task-applied dramatherapy include:

- more confidence in their own acceptability to others; an increased sense of being valuable in themselves

- greater awareness of the ways they themselves react to other people, and of the particular circumstances which are associated with whatever it may be about themselves that they want to change

- actual experience of having behaved in ways that they usually believe either difficult or impossible to achieve.

This last is the crucial element in all behavioural change. It does not belong only to dramatherapy. What is special here is the awareness of personal safety, within a setting specifically designed to create such feelings, and consequently the increased sense of freedom and possibility which comes from experimenting with new kinds of personal relationship which suggest alternative ways of behaving towards other people and interpreting their behaviour towards oneself – in other words, the dramatherapy session used as a laboratory for experiments in relationship, rather than a classroom where people are taught how to interact with one another.

The most important thing of all, the fact that distinguishes drama-therapy from other approaches, is the reality of these new kinds of experiences. Although such dramatherapy sessions are 'staged', in the sense of largely depending on a set of procedures planned in advance and the establishment of a carefully contrived atmosphere of safety combined with stimulation, the interpersonal experiences they give rise to are completely genuine, in the sense of being natural and unforced. There is no suggestion here of changing behaviour 'from the outside in'. The people who find themselves thinking, feeling and behaving in ways they previously considered 'unimaginable' remain conscious of having experienced and benefited from something which was not simply a kind of training for life but a genuine episode in the history of their relationships with other people, a real part of life itself. Whereas much of what is done in the name of psychological healing takes place 'behind the scenes', clinically separated from the ordinary life of patients and clients, dramatherapy has the ability to focus our awareness on the real thing, happening here and now within our ongoing life stories. Its subject matter is not isolated behaviours painstakingly detached from the men, women and children they belong to, but things done and said by whole people, persons-in-relation engaged in the all-absorbing process of maximising their wholeness.

In fact, the focus of task-applied dramatherapy is on wholeness, the interpersonal event in its entirety, not distorted or exaggerated or with parts sectioned off for closer scrutiny. Disturbed behaviour is remedied by working towards the restoration of balance in the ways that individuals react to real social situations rather than simply aiming at the replacement of one fixed pattern of behaviour by another. This basic attitude to healing is the source of dramatherapy's generalisability as a treatment modality – the reason why it is so useful in a range of different applications.

Some applications of task-applied dramatherapy are given here. Each session is divided into three parts:

- warm-up
- main activity
- closure.

## Social skills 1

*Warm-up*

- Group members stand near the walls of the room, facing the wall. Ask people to check whether they feel too close to another person. If so, move and find a place where they feel more comfortable. Stand very close to the wall, then move away taking a few steps backwards or turning to move away and then turning back to the wall. Focus on a mark, pattern or object on the wall, study it and notice the components of the whole. Move forward and stand very close to the wall. Focus on the chosen site again and study the site chosen. Become aware of the difference between viewing in the two places. Now move and find the place which gives you the best view of the object or mark.

*Discussion: how far away did people need to be in order to gain the best overall view? Group members are invited to show others the positions they found.*

- Stand near to walls again but facing away from the wall. Stand with back against the wall. Move so that parts of the back of the body make contact with the wall. Start to involve hands and arms. With feet remaining in one position make contact with the wall with as many parts of the body as possible. Make sure no discomfort is caused. Relax and move a few steps away from the wall. Re-create the position created when in contact with the wall. Relax. Shake arms and legs.

- Continue with shaking movements. Imagine that the body is like a string puppet and start to change these movements into the kind of movement a puppet might make. Continue with these movements and start to move around the room.

*Discussion: how did these different movements feel?*

*Main activity*

- Move to different parts of the room. Focus on a point some distance from you. Start to move towards that place. Stop. Become aware that other people may cross your path. If you meet someone on your way, stop and negotiate a way around them without speaking. Continue on your way to your point in the room. Stand still when you reach your point and wait until everyone else is in place. Repeat, moving towards another point in the room.

- Focus on another point in the room, this time on the wall. Focus on the point and stand a little more upright. This time when you meet another person, stand facing them and make eye contact for a few seconds before moving on to your focused point.

- As before, but this time making eye contact. Say 'excuse me' each time you have made it.

*Discussion: on the space needed between people when they meet.*

*Closure*

- Brainstorm circumstances in which people might say 'excuse me', i.e. situations where we might need to pass people or move around them.

- Dramatise the situation, taking time to set the scene and allow different people to become the person who says 'excuse me'. You may need to 'freeze' the action when the words are spoken, to explore the appropriate actions for the people the request is made to. It is sometimes useful to do these exercises in slow motion after the first attempt, i.e. an 'action replay' for any observers to comment upon. How were the movements made? What made them effective? In what way was eye contact made? How did it affect interaction? If the group is really unable to provide any examples, use some that have been prepared.

*Focus of group: spatial relationships; becoming aware of different parts of the body; speech and body co-ordination.*

## Social skills 2

*Warm-up*

- Walk freely around the room, noticing other people. Maybe say 'hello' as you pass. Start to walk slightly faster and notice the clothes other people are wearing. Notice colour, fabric and style. Which are nearest to the clothes you are wearing? Start to make verbal contact with other people. Comment on the similarities between the items they are wearing and your own attire. The similarities may be colour, shape, fabric or style. Meet as many people as possible. Sometimes it may take a while to find the similarities between you.

- *Game.* 'The sun shines on …' Stand or sit in a circle. If sitting, there should be one chair fewer than the number of people in the group. One person stands in the middle of the circle and says 'The sun shines on everyone who …' (for example) 'is wearing something yellow', 'had cornflakes for breakfast', 'likes walking' or whatever. Everyone who relates to what is said moves to a vacated chair in the space left by someone else. The person who does not find a space is the next person to be in the centre. Change the ways in which people move; for example, in slow motion or hopping. If using fast movements ensure that safety is maintained.

- Remain in a circle. The group leaders stand in the middle of the circle and ask participants to make the circle larger. The leaders ask group members to close their eyes. While eyes are closed the leaders adopt a particular posture. Participants are asked to mirror the shapes created by the leaders. (As they are in a circle they will all get a slightly different view of the shape.) Repeat several times.

*Discussion: how did it feel to reproduce a shape that someone else had created? What was the same as your familiar posture and what was different?*

*Main activity*

- Group members stand in a circle. One person stands in the centre and makes the shape of someone looking sad. Other group members may make suggestions about the posture. Once a posture has been established, other group members are invited, one by one, to enter the centre of the circle and make a gesture which is a response to the 'sculpture' of sadness. This is done silently and held for a number of seconds. Repeat with different group members taking up postures of other emotions.

*Discussion: after each emotion has been shown and responded to, discuss the different approaches which felt appropriate.*

- Repeat the above format but this time, in pairs, add a few words. (Group leaders may need to have some emotions written on pieces of paper to hand out to the pairs.) The pairs show their sculptures to the rest of the group.

*Discussion: how did the posture and the words complement each other?*

- Set chairs in horseshoe shape with one chair in the centre of the gap.
- Brainstorm the ways in which we might indicate to other people that we are not willing to be approached or spoken to. For example, arms and legs crossed with closed posture or 'hiding behind a newspaper'. Group members are asked to try out some of the postures, sitting on or standing behind the central chair. As each person demonstrates, others comment on the way signals are being conveyed.
- Place another chair by the side of the single chair. One person sits on one of these chairs in a position that conveys that he or she is willing to be approached. As the previous exercise has demonstrated 'closed' body posture, this one will show an 'open' body posture. If a person is finding it difficult to adopt a posture, brainstorm to find out the reason. Once posture is established, invite another group member to sit in the empty chair and find a further posture which will indicate they are willing to engage in conversation. When everyone who wants to has taken a turn, discuss the levels of communication shown.
- Brainstorm topics of conversation we have when we meet people. Think back to game at start of group, i.e. 'similarities between people'. In pairs, create scenarios using the types of

posture explored above. Person A takes time to create a posture and person B responds. This time add speech. Repeat, alternating roles of A and B.

*Discussion: on general experience of combining speech and movement.*

*Closure*

- Divide into two groups. Group 1 adopt the postures of wanting to communicate; people from group 2 approach them and tell them about what they have enjoyed about their contribution to today's group. Reverse roles.
- Goodbyes, and close group.

*Focus of group: self and other(s). How do I show how I feel about sharing?*

## Social skills 3

*Equipment: large sheets of paper, A4 paper, felt-tipped pens.*

*Warm-up*

- Group members walk around the room:
  - (a) looking at the floor
  - (b) looking straight ahead
  - (c) noticing other people and acknowledging them by eye contact
  - (d) making some appropriate physical contact: handshakes, a hand on shoulder.

*Discussion: on appropriate touch.*

*Main activity*

- Using a very large sheet of paper, either have a body outline prepared or ask a volunteer to lie down on the paper and then draw round the person. Group members sit around the shape on the paper and discuss the areas of the body that are appropriate for touch in different situations.

*Questions:*

(a)  What are the differences between touch from/to friends, family, strangers, children, older people? Are there gender differences?

(b)  What are the public/private areas of the body? Use felt-tipped pens to make a map. (It may be useful for each person to have an A4 size body outline to mark with different colours.)

(c)  In pairs, demonstrate the different touch relationships between different pairs of characters (e.g. mother–daughter, salesperson–customer, older person–child, friends). Are there some of these where touch is not appropriate?

*Closure*

• Group members invent different ways of saying goodbye to one another. Close group.

*Focus of group: appropriate and inappropriate touch.*

## Social skills 4

*Warm-up*

• Collect hats, music, mirrors. *Game.* Participants sit in a circle. Hats are distributed, and everyone tries on their hat. They create a posture appropriate to the hat. Group leader plays music and the hats are passed around the circle in time to the music. When the music is stopped each person places the hat they are holding on their head and adopts the relevant posture. Repeat several times.

• Put hats into the centre of the circle or on a table. Participants each choose a hat and place it on their head, using a mirror to view themselves. They walk around the room in the way that a person wearing this hat might do. How is this affected by shoes, dress, one's opinion of oneself? When group members have experimented with walks, they greet each other in the manner of the character.

- What kind of environment would this person be found in? Will this be inside or outside? Is it a hot or cold place? Create these environments in different areas of the room.

*Main activity*

- Divide into pairs. Person A (out of role) tells Person B about his or her character and its environment. Person A assumes the role of B's character and enters their environment. Person B enters as themselves and interviews the person. Allow 5–7 minutes. Reverse roles in exercise. Form different pairs and repeat.

*Discussion: on the relationships and the social interaction. How were the interactions affected by culture, race, gender, class, ability, disability?*

*Closure*

- Group members say goodbye to one another in the way they are most used to doing. Close group.

*Focus of group: status and social interaction.*

## Social skills 5

*Warm-up*

- Walk round the room, recognising people and saying hello to them.
- Walk round room mentioning to people you meet times when you have been together before.

*Main activity*

- Walk round again. This time one person wears a cloak or a similar item which distinguishes them from other people. It is suggested that this person is 'different' from everyone else in the group. How might people react when passing them? People take turns to wear the distinguishing item.

*Discussion: on the differences between people. Are there some things about people that make them different? Is it fair to say this is different?*

- In groups of three or four, create scenarios in which one person is 'different'. Prepare two short pieces of drama to show to the other group. The first piece shows people behaving rudely and thoughtlessly to the isolated person. The second piece shows equality.

*Closure*

- Discuss in relation to social interactions. What is it like to meet together in a group like this?
- Say goodbye, and close the group.

*Focus of group: on differences between people. How to interact when meeting someone who may appear different. Exploring prejudice.*

*Note:* For people wishing to work in a dramatic way with social skills training, Johnstone (1981) contains valuable chapters on status and improvisational skills.

## Anger management 1

*Warm-up*

- Ask people to say who they are.
- Everyone says hello to the group as a whole, and then spends a moment talking to somebody else.

*Main activity*

- Participants seated in a circle. Imagine your anger as an object. Consider whether it is heavy, light, sticky, smooth, spiked or of some other texture. How would it feel to hold this object? (If people have created large objects, ask them to imagine that they have shrunk and can be held in the hands.) Hold the imaginary object in both hands and experiment with moving the object to points at various distances away from the body.

- Hold the object as if it is a ball. Start to throw and catch it while remaining seated. Leave chairs and throw and catch 'ball' while walking around the room. Stop and think about childhood and adult ball games.

- Each person declares the game they have thought of. Set the scene and play each game. (For example, someone has volunteered snooker. Select the players and the observers. Where will they stand? Are the observers supporting the players or are they passive? The person who chose the game explains the rules and something about the properties of the ball. Which colour is it? Is it a standard snooker ball or will it retain some of the properties given to it?) Give people time to play all of the games or divide the group into two and play two games simultaneously.

*Discussion: consider the rules of the game. Are there real-life games that are played out involving anger? What rules could provide boundaries? What is uncomfortable about the game? What part of the game needs to be changed? What rules could be created?*

*Closure*

- What was it like making up games together? Tell someone about it one-to-one.
- Say goodbye to this person, then to the group.

*Focus of group: controlled anger by the use of projective structures; allowing us to control the anger rather than be controlled by it.*

## Anger management 2

*Equipment: paper, felt-tipped pens.*

*Warm-up*

- Participants walk around the room. Become aware of the way your body moves. Focus on the connections between different body parts. How does movement change when different parts of the body lead the movement? Try being 'led' by your shoulders, hips, knees, hands.

*Discussion: how did it feel to have different parts of the body leading movement?*

*Main activity*

- Consider the body sensations that lead up to anger. Isolate the very first sensation. Each person draws a graph which charts the way that the sensations build to inappropriate anger. Which body parts lead during the display of anger? Which parts become suppressed or inactive? For example, the throat can become too tight to produce sound or any verbal expressions of anger.

- In a sitting or standing position create a frozen posture or 'sculpt' of the final image on the graph, i.e. the body. Show the body in action during a display of anger. Move to another chair or position in the room and make a sculpt of the parts of the body which are not in action. (The whole body will represent this part.) Move between these two positions.

*Discussion: what is it like allowing your body to express feelings?*

*Closure*

- Each person has two sheets of paper, headed with the names of two body parts. For example, one sheet could be headed 'fists', the other 'throat'. Write a list of words that describe the state that part is in during a bout of anger. Example:

| *Throat* | *Fists* |
|---|---|
| tight | clenched |
| constricted | out of control |
| controlled | tense |
| wanting to speak | damaging |

- When participants have completed this list, write a dialogue between the two parts. Example:

    *Throat*: I want to be heard but I am too constricted. Please listen to me.

    *Fists*:  We are too busy just now. We are out of control.

    *Throat*: Stop for a moment and let me breathe.

- Complete the dialogue by allowing the throat to speak and achieve a relaxed state. The fists, too, become relaxed. (*Adaptations: focus on internal organs, e.g. the heart versus the guts, or on different states of mind, e.g. reason versus emotion.*) It is possible to create a drama from the scripts and share it with other group members.

*Focus of group: creating your own rules to manage anger. How allowing attention to be paid to the body can change the stimuli for action in anger.*

## Assertiveness training

Here are some suggestions to be used in a similar kind of format: warm-up, main activity and closure.

Assertiveness can be viewed as aiming to achieve balance in our lives. Being passive, aggressive or indirectly aggressive makes us out of balance with ourselves and other people. As dramatherapy works towards an integration of the body and mind, the following are examples that may be included in the early stages of a dramatherapy-based assertiveness training group.

*Balance – sitting in chairs (Activities 1–6)*

ACTIVITY 1

- Back supported by chair back. Feet uncrossed and flat on floor. Become aware of the way in which the chair supports your weight. Shift position several times and become aware of the effect of changing from a comfortable position to an uncomfortable position. Become aware of tension in your body and the feelings this tension produces.

*Discussion: the discomfort of being in an unbalanced position. Draw links between being in an unbalanced interaction with someone else. For example, when you say yes when you want to say no, when you feel let down but say 'it's OK', or when you let out a rush of angry words when you want to be treated fairly.*

ACTIVITY 2

- Feet on floor, legs uncrossed, hands on lap, palms down. Become aware of breathing. Slowly deepen breathing without creating any tension in the body. If possible, breathe in and out of the nose. Breathe in for a count of four and out to a count of four. Slowly take the breath deeper and deeper into the body. Pause for a count of one before exhaling and next inhalation.

*Discussion: feel the difference between shallow and deep breathing. This standard relaxation exercise can be repeated regularly throughout the group.*

ACTIVITY 3A

- In chairs without arms. Start by sitting with feet on the floor and back supported by chair back. Change position and focus on the amount of space the body takes up on the chair. Change positions alternating between taking up a lot of space and as little space as possible.

*Discussion: relate the positions to the behaviour types outlined in assertiveness training manuals. When we are aggressive we take up too much space; in passive behaviour we take up too little space. Explore these issues literally and metaphorically. Assertiveness means taking enough space for ourselves and allowing enough for others.*

ACTIVITY 3B

This is a continuation of activity 3A. Put three armless chairs together in a line.

- In pairs. First each person takes up as little space as possible. Try several positions. Then each person takes up as much space as possible. Nominate Person A and Person B. Person A takes up a large amount of space; B takes up a small amount of space. Try several variations, then change roles.

*Discussion: discuss how doing this exercise felt. Relate to assertiveness. Which were the most familiar positions for people?*

ACTIVITY 3C

- Find ways of both taking up the same amount of space so the chosen positions feel comfortable for both partners.

*Discussion: discuss all three parts of this activity.*

ACTIVITY 4

- Set chairs to face each other. Each person sits in a chair, so that two rows of people face each other. One row of people close their eyes and the other row take up a position that involves leaning forward. They make an outward gesture with arms and hands that reach into their partners' space. For example, this can be an aggressive gesture or a pleading gesture. When postures are set the other row of people open their eyes and make a gesture in response. Repeat several times. Change roles.

*Discussion: discuss feelings engendered. It is helpful to do this activity in the rows rather than in pairs around the room as this grouping can add focus and aid concentration. Other people are also in view and their gestures may have meaning for people other than their partner.*

ACTIVITY 5

- 'The chair on my right is free.' This well-known drama game can also be adapted to emphasise the behaviour types. A circle of chairs is set out, one for each group member and one empty chair. The person with the empty chair on the right says, 'The chair on my right is free and I would like [*person's name*] to sit in it.' The named person moves to the empty chair, creating another empty chair in the circle. The person with this chair on their right repeats the above phrase and the named person moves. Repeat five or six times. Now ask people to repeat the phrase 'The chair on my right etc.' in a passive manner. Make sure that most people have spoken, then change to aggressive demands; indirectly aggressive; and finally assertive.

*Discussion: discuss the differences in voice tone and movement. This exercise can also be useful later in the group when the subject is 'giving and receiving compliments'. The phrase is completed with 'because' and a compliment about the person requested to move. The person moving responds by saying, 'Thank you, I am pleased you like...'*

ACTIVITY 6

- Place chairs in a circle with spaces between them. Each person sits in a chair and makes themselves comfortable. Individuals look around the circle and notice other people, making eye contact and acknowledging the person they have made eye contact with in a non-verbal way. Allow five minutes to discuss how this contact felt.

The exercises in chairs have introduced the concepts of space and balance and are useful in sessions 1–3. During sessions 3–4, group members should feel ready to leave their chairs. If not, continue with chair work and gradually move into standing position. Use exercises which include finding different ways to leave the chair, using an out-breath to pull the body into a standing position, using arms to pull body forward and out of the chair. Work with different parts of the body to take the lead from sitting to standing position.

*Balance – standing up (Activities 7–9)*

ACTIVITY 7

- Find your own space in the room. Stand with feet firmly on the ground, slightly apart. Move feet until body is in a balanced position. Breathe deeply and slowly. Imagine a colour that you connect with balance. Imagine breathing in this colour and allow it to very gently make a smooth line through your body, dividing at your hips and running through your legs. Very gently allow the line of colour to make your body feel slightly taller. Allow the colour to fill your body with confidence. Now shift your body into a retreating, passive stance and again find a colour and repeat the first exercise. Repeat, finding different colours for anger, aggression and manipulative behaviour. Discuss the differences in feelings using these postures.

*Discussion: relate the first feeling of balance to assertive behaviour.*

ACTIVITY 8

- Stand with a partner, facing each other, and divide into A and B. A starts to make soft, flowing movements with hands and arms. B responds with the same type of movement. Continue until the whole body is moving. Start to move, in pairs, around the room. Repeat using (a) jagged, angular movements, (b) harsh, punching movements, (c) one person using strong pushing movements as other person retreats.

*Discussion: relate the movements to assertive, passive and aggressive modes of behaviour. What were the feelings aroused? This exercise can also include mirroring and/or be done to music.*

ACTIVITY 9

- Stand in a circle, with enough space between people for arms to be stretched out to the side. Each person stands with feet apart in a balanced position: (a) gently stretch arms to 'claim space', gently touching fingers of next person; (b) thrust arms out to claim space; (c) very tentatively claim space with arms.

*Discussion: discuss in relation to assertively claiming 'our own space'.*

These activities have touched on spatial relationship. Activity 10 extends this area.

ACTIVITY 10

- Group members stand in a row at one end of the room. One person stands facing them at the other end of the room. One by one, people leave the row and walk towards the single person. This person says 'stop' when they feel that the person approaching them is too close. (If this is not said in a convincing manner, people continue to approach.) Repeat until everyone has had a turn. If facing a row of people is too daunting the exercise can be done in pairs. As participants engage in the exercise remind them of the balance and breathing exercises.

- In pairs, one person sitting in a chair facing front. Their partner approaches them and stands to their side. The person in the chair uses breathing exercises and balance to maintain an assertive posture even though they are in the more vulnerable position. Practise with person standing taking different positions around chair. Then reverse roles. This exercise can also be done with (a) one person behind a desk; (b) one person holding papers and 'hiding behind them'. Ask participants for other power-based positions. The aim of the exercises is to aid participants to maintain balance and be assertive when they seem to be at a physical disadvantage.

## Rights

(This is to be used in the threefold dramatherapy format.)

Ask group to provide a list of the rights they believe human beings have. Discuss which of these are genuinely rights. For example, do we have the right to respect or is it something to be earned? (Phelps and Austin's (1988) book on assertiveness training provides guidelines.)

ACTIVITY 1

- Form a circle. One person outlines a right they find difficult to believe in. They then stand in front of each individual in the circle and express their entitlement to the chosen right. The person they are speaking to denies them that right. This is then reclaimed by the person expressing the right. For example:

  A group member is struggling with the right to say no without feeling guilty. They stand in the middle of the circle and take time to adjust their breathing to deep slow breaths and to put their body into their position of balance. Once they feel 'balanced', they stand facing the other group member. They say, 'I have the right to say no without feeling guilty.' The person facing them says, 'No – you do not have the right to say no without guilt.' They then reply, 'Yes I do have the right to say no without feeling guilty.' Repeat around the circle so this group member speaks to every person in the group. (*Note:* It is important that the chosen right is repeated, in full, during every interaction as this confirms the right. Some group members may need another person, maybe one of the group leaders, to accompany them on the journey around the group. This person may prompt but should remain silent, providing support by their presence only.)

*Discussion: angry feelings engendered by exercise after everyone has completed. This activity may provoke strong emotional feelings so allow at least a quarter of an hour to process.*

ACTIVITY 2

Each group member decides on the rights that are most relevant to them. Each one makes a list and is then offered the opportunity to participate in the following exercise.

- A space is cleared at one end of the room. One person enters this space and reads out their list of rights. She or he then asks other group members to 'become these rights' (one per person). One by one the other group members are invited into the space with the words 'I welcome the right to [*insert right*] into my life.' The protagonist literally welcomes the person representing the right into the space (the form of welcome will depend on the level of touch people are confident with). Once the right has been welcomed its 'owner' provides some examples of how she or he will use it. This is said directly to the person representing the right. 'You are the right to [*insert name of right*] and I will use you to…' Each person is invited to be the protagonist.

*Discussion: discuss ways that these rights will enhance the quality of the participants' lives. Facilitators do not need to focus on how the important issues are about the personal ownership of rights.*

*Needs and wants*

(This is to be used in the threefold dramatherapy format.)

ACTIVITY 1

- Each person has a large sheet of paper and some felt-tipped pens. At the top of the sheet the word 'WANT' is written. People write 'I want…' in large print under this. Brainstorm words and sayings directly and indirectly connected with these two words. Recall childhood experiences of saying 'I want' and the responses from adults.

*Discussion: how have taboos on saying 'I want' been carried into adult life?*

ACTIVITY 2

- Group members seated in circle. What kind of movements are associated with 'I want'? (For example, foot stamping, clenched fists, frowning.) Relate 'I want' to assertiveness training. Each member stands in the centre of a circle, finds position of balance and states 'I want' several times in an even tone.

*Discussion: discuss the effect of hearing 'I want' said in an assertive manner. Discuss the difference between 'I want' and 'I need'.*

*Consolidation*

All of the activities can now be brought together for role rehearsals of life situations. Encourage group members to provide examples of situations where they find it difficult to be assertive.

To prepare for a dramatisation of the particular situation, consider the following:

*Who?*

Give careful thought to who it is that you want this action plan to focus on.

*What?*

Be very specific about what it is that you want and try to phrase this positively. We often find it easier to think about what we DO NOT want, but assertiveness is about asking honestly, openly and clearly for what we DO want and need.

*What are my rights?*

Examine the situation carefully to see which of your rights is being taken away – or you are giving away. Also remember that the other person also has rights and you should think about how those relate to the situation. This is usually the basis for some compromise to be achieved.

*What are my thoughts and feelings?*

If you spend some time examining both of these then you should have a clearer idea of what may be preventing you from acting assertively. Owning up to – and owning – our own thoughts and feelings can be hard work, but it is a good way to prepare for acting assertively.

*When?*

Think about timing – it can make all the difference!

*Where?*

Also important. If you can have some choice over time and place then you will feel more confident.

*How?*

Remember the assertive way: open, honest and direct (try to keep it short and simple, too).

# CHAPTER 3

# The Creative-Expressive Mode

## Dramatherapy and Role

'I propose[d] the theory that the child's play is the infantile form of the human ability to deal with experience by creating model situations and to master reality by experiment and planning' (Erikson 1965, p.214). In Chapter 2 we glanced at the usefulness of playing games in dramatherapy. For human beings game playing (in the literal sense; we shall be mentioning the less literal one later) is not simply useful, it is fundamental. It builds worlds.

The urge to play is an original characteristic of the entire human species. It is psycho-formative; in other words, the way we put our minds together. Peter Slade (1995) describes two basic forms of child play: 'projected' and 'personal'. In *projected* play 'the body is mostly still ... and the idea, or dream in their mind, is projected into, onto or around objects outside them. "Life" is going on in the objects during this activity, and there may be strong emotion or love or importance associated with them' (Slade 1995, p.2). When he talks of playthings having a life of their own, he is describing the phenomenon that Winnicott (1971) calls the 'transitional object', the treasured personal possession – 'a bundle of wood or the corner of a blanket or eiderdown, or a word or a line or a mannerism' (Winnicott 1971, p.115) – which a child uses to bridge the vital gap between self and environment and 'give life to the world'. Slade points out that the distinctive feature of this kind of playing is that it makes a definite mark on the world in the shape of tangible evidence that it has been going on: '...the things played with remain as a memorial, a monument of their doing' (Slade 1995, p.2).

*Personal* play, on the other hand, involves the whole person who 'gets up and moves about and takes total physical, emotional or spiritual responsibility for the action. No longer can the toy or doll live life for you,

you are now up and doing it yourself' (Slade 1995, p.3). This play is dance, movement and drama, in which we ourselves move out into the world instead of sending a messenger ahead of us in order to try out the lie of the land on our behalf. At least this is what we may seem to be doing. In fact, a little observation should tell us that this kind of playing, like projected play, also depends upon imagination, and is in fact itself a kind of transitional activity. We may provide ourselves with functional explanations for the enjoyment we get from running, dancing, skating, even doing exercises to tone up our muscles and shape our abdomens, but as soon as we give these activities any kind of imaginative framework, even if this is simply enjoying the idea of winning a race or looking really slim, they become for us a kind of projected game. (If you doubt this, try flexing your muscles in the mirror!) In fact, imagination makes everything – even work itself – into a game; and imagination is indispensable if you want to be human!

Writing from a psychoanalytic point of view, Erikson (1965) regards games as playing a functional role for adults as well as children, and describes how imagination provides a blueprint for action in the world.

> It is in certain phases of his work that the adult projects past experience into dimensions which seem manageable. In the laboratory, on the stage and on the drawing board, he relives the past and thus relieves left over effects; in re-constructing the model situation he redeems his failures and strengthens his hopes. (Erikson 1965, pp.214–215)

With children, so with adults: the purpose of play is to create *courage*. Armed with our blueprint, the product of all our exercises in trying life out for size, we step forth into the real world ready to face its challenges, whether they are practical, emotional or both. They are always *relational*, because they always concern our relationship with whatever is not our self. The courage we need is the courage to face life as individual persons in society, and this, as Rollo May (1975) points out, is closely linked to creativity: 'Creative courage is the discovery of new forms, new symbols, new patterns, on which the new society can be built' (May 1975, p.21). For child and adult alike, play is workshop, laboratory, studio – the place and time for imagination to forge a creative response to life.

Herein lies the difference between the two ways in which we use the verb 'to play': first, to describe what a child or adult does, either alone or in company, when they are involved in a game of some kind; second, to describe somebody actually taking part in *a play*, a piece of theatre. The link between the two ideas, and the reason why we use the word associated with games to describe the business of pretending to be someone else in an actual, acted, drama, is very straightforward. The one is simply an extension of the other (see Wickham 1959). We use our ability to play games as the raw material of theatre. And so we play in both places, on the stage and in the garden or nursery, using our native ability to remember and live within a framework of imagination. This is why we do not tell people whom we meet that we are 'performing a drama', or 'taking part in a stage production'; what we say is, 'I'm in a play.' Whether they take place in the school playground or on the stage of the Royal Shakespeare Theatre, our games possess the same content. They are an imaginative reconstruction of experience.

Constantin Stanislavski, the greatest twentieth-century teacher of actors, speaks of 'emotional memory' (1948), stressing the way in which an actor uses his or her own personal life-experience to give genuine human reality to 'characters' whose 'life' is otherwise simply an idea confined to the imagination of somebody reading a play-script. For Stanislavski an actor's experience is the raw material out of which the actor will create the new, imagined person alive in the world of the play – as children make use of what they know and have lived through in order to explore things they do not know but can imagine. Theatre itself consists of sharing an imaginative game in which author, actors and audience are all 'principals' because each of them contributes to the play as a whole event. The fact is underlined by the work of Bertolt Brecht, who stresses the game-like nature of the proceedings and the freedom of the audience to decide that they do not want to play the game according to the rules set out for them by the characters in the drama.

This game-like, fun quality of theatre is an important part of drama-therapy, whose aim is not to manipulate people's awareness, but to find ways of co-operating with them in giving reality to the things they dare imagine, the characters they choose to create. Thus it aims at being a game, not a technique. In the kind of playing which comes under the general heading of 'enactment', personal and projected play are united in a single experience, as the self presents its own life to other people, and also, at the same time, to itself. The idea of enactment is central to dramatherapy simply because it lies at the very heart of the way that women and men manage the business of being alive, being human. As Sue Jennings (1990) puts it, in dramatherapy we remind ourselves of something we often overlook, and may even have forgotten altogether; we can test our behaviour out before 'playing it for real', a fact of life on which our basic socialisation depends.

This is how Jennings describes the growing child's introduction to the dramatic processes which she or he will be involved in as a normal, natural part of living: 'From birth to a year old the child is involved in a variety of explorations of the senses. It can make sounds and rhythms, it can make marks (albeit with food and faeces), and it can imitate' (Jennings 1990, p.14). This is the time of growing awareness of the expressive potential of possessing a body, what Jennings calls the *embodiment* stage. However, the child does not stop there, of course:

> Once the infant is finger painting and playing with toys and objects outside itself, it is moving from the embodiment stage of experience to the *projective* stage. Experiences are played out and discovered through media outside the infant; for example, the feelings associated with making a mess or pouring water. Dramatic play then develops through situational dramatic events from real life, stories and fairy tales. (Jennings 1990, p.14)

Consequently the child moves into Jennings' third stage, the most explicitly dramatic of all as 'the infant starts to take on *roles*, playing many parts and changing voices' (Jennings 1990, p.14).

'One man in his time plays many parts' – and starts doing it very early indeed. Most of the time, of course, we remain unconscious of the intricate social dramas in which we are involved, experiencing it in Mary Duggan's words as a 'seamless matrix of action and interaction where figure and ground are in constant flux; where actors and audience are one' (Duggan and Grainger 1997, p.54). We are so used to this state of affairs we tend to regard ourselves as totally bound by its rules as if we were completely locked into our own role. Whether we choose to play a particular part in life or not, we regard ourselves as 'stuck' with it and in it, seeing it as part of ourselves, as inevitable as eye-colour or country of origin. Certainly the demands of belonging within a particular family or social network are strict enough; we must somehow perform our own role with close regard to the performance of the rest of the cast or the play will fall apart so far as we are concerned. What we often forget, however (what we need to be reminded about), is that although this system of action and reaction certainly exists we ourselves have more influence over it than we think we do. If we have each developed the ability, first of all to see ourselves playing different roles, and then to go ahead and play these roles, we have therefore the power to alter, to a greater or lesser degree, the plot of the whole social drama. *And we do have this power.* What we need is the wisdom and discretion to use it to our own and other people's best advantage; the wisdom, the discretion and *the confidence.*

Dramatherapy is not so much for developing skill as gaining confidence; not so much the confidence to play a particular role better than we did before (although it can help us do that), more the confidence to see ourselves as genuinely in charge of our role-playing and not subject to other people's ideas about what roles are available or suitable for us to inhabit. As masters of our own role-playing we are able, if we want to, to change the roles we find ourselves playing. In other words it is about becoming more flexible as *actors* – in the Shakespearean sense of the word – and more resilient as *people*, in every sense of the word. It is about feeling more free, more responsible and more in charge of our own lives. A basic purpose of dramatherapy, then, is to help us gain more control of our own role-playing, the ways in which we enact our relationship with ourselves and other people who, to a greater or lesser degree, constitute our personal world. Through acting out who we are, we enlarge our vision of the people we are capable of being, using the freedom dramatherapy gives us to be all sorts of selves, all kinds of people, as a rehearsal for our life 'on the stage of the world'. Thus through enactment and re-enactment those taking part are encouraged to re-invest in the fundamental human ability to maintain their social identity.

The fact that social life itself is organised as if it were a play has been studied intensively by Erving Goffman, by examining the actual behaviour of individuals and groups in ordinary 'real life' social situations and noting the kinds of things they do and say in order to sustain their performances (Goffman 1990). Goffman is a sociologist: for him 'all the world's a stage' is primarily a sociological metaphor, a useful way of looking at how the social world is organised, drawing on all the evidence provided by the correspondence between various social institutions and accepted kinds of interpersonal behaviour, and the way theatre 'works'. (For example, the systematic relationship which exists between 'on-stage', 'off-stage' and 'back-stage' in the arrangements that individuals and communities make for living together.)

Goffman is associated with the idea of role-distance. Individuals are not to be wholly identified with the role they play as if they actually *were* that role, and not a person who for one reason or another has assumed it and, for the time being, feels he or she has to keep on playing it. However, when the person feels that the time is ripe, one 'social mask' may be cast aside and another taken up, or as is more likely in situations concerning actual human beings, the person concerned may embark on a more or less gradual process of involving the transfer of role identity. This, too, is obviously an idea taken from the theatre. As such, it has been considerably extended and deepened by Robert Landy (1993), working from the evidence provided by actual plays written for and presented in the theatre. With great subtlety and insight, Landy analyses the distinctive characteristics of the personages who appear on stage in the dramatic literature of the world, in order to arrive at a catalogue of available dramatic roles and discover what it is that allows a role to make dramatic sense, as someone we can recognise as the kind of person we have either actually met or can imagine ourselves meeting. In other words, we are helped to understand the world we live in by recognising the roles people play in it, and helped to recognise these roles by reading plays and going to the theatre.

The reason why these theatrical roles stand out as actual people, 'personages', each distinguishable in their own right, is that we can somehow recognise their uniqueness. These play-people are both like us and different from us at the same time. They are individuals before being types, just like the people we know. The author has created them to be people, to be *themselves*; and that is what makes them alive for us, able to strike chords in our experience, both in real life and fantasy, although we may sometimes be at a loss to say which particular chords it is that are resonating. It is certainly not simply a case of having 'met somebody like that' or 'been in this sort of group'. Somehow, these stage characters whom we have never met before make sense to us; because they are recognisable they have the effect of making life more recognisable for us. Landy (1993) sets out not to categorise particular types, but to catalogue the range of human roles remembered and imagined by playwrights throughout the world. Whether this is feasible in any final sense is open to question, of course. Certainly he does not claim that his own list is exclusive; what it does do, very powerfully, is draw attention to the vital importance of theatre and drama as ways of understanding what is involved in being human.

Human roles represent the parts we play in life. Acted roles, either improvised or written down in plays, make human role-playing clear and explicit. When people speak about 'role-playing' they tend not to mean what happens in real plays, however. What they mean is pretending to be somebody you are not. This is the cross that drama bears in our culture – to be perpetually associated with the intention of deceiving people. When we consider the use of masks in dramatherapy in Chapter 4 we shall be looking at this more closely. For the time being, however, it should simply be pointed out that without our natural impulse to take on a role, and to change that role according to the circumstances we find ourselves in, we should simply not be human at all: not because we would be prevented from deceiving people but because we would find ourselves without the ability to enter into any kind of relationship with them at all, and if we could we would not be able to sustain it. Our role is the way in which we present ourselves to other people. It is the way we present ourselves to ourselves. It is about living and dying in the presence of others. We may play it insincerely, hiding our real thoughts and feelings, our true selves, behind it. This side of role-playing has been well documented (see Jourard 1964; Winnicott 1960), perhaps because it is the side that gives us most trouble as well as attracting almost all the attention. As well as being the most painful aspect of role-playing it is also the most obvious. Most of our roles are so genuine, so much ourselves that nobody really recognises them as roles because they are part of us, and it is us that people see. Only when we are using them as a defensive ploy, without letting on that we are doing so, do they become obvious to others. This is because there is a kind of gap between oneself and the role one is playing, so its nature as a role, something we are hiding behind, is quite apparent.

The following examples of dramatherapy practice are concerned with self-preservation and finding one's role among other people as oneself. In order to find this role, these processes will include methods of experimenting with dramatic characters. This is a 12-week group structure.

## Session 1

- Group members warm up by introducing themselves to each other, giving their names.

*Group rules and group culture*

- Move slowly around the room, noticing the colours of items around the room. Notice the way that the lighting may create bright areas and shadows.
- Find small items that are of your favourite colour. Bring one of these items with you to a seated circle of group members and facilitators.
- Discuss the colours and the differences that light and shade make to the item. What connections can be made with the chosen colours? (These may be personal or scenic. For example, 'Blue reminds me of a clear sky or a calm sea.')
- Remain in the circle. Notice the colours that people are wearing. In turn, make verbal connections with each other based on shared colours. Devise a format that is in keeping with the general ability of the group. Check the names of the group members at the same time as making connections through colour.
- Finish the session with a general discussion about how colour affects people on a day-to-day basis. Depart after saying goodbye to everyone in the group by exchanging handshakes.

*Purpose: to become familiar with other group members and the environment. To introduce the theme of colour and the importance of colour in everyday life.*

## Session 2

*Warm-up*

- Form a standing circle. Each person shakes hands with the person to the left and then with the person to the right, giving a

greeting at the same time as the handshake. This can be verbal
or non-verbal; for example, a spoken hello or a smile.

- Each person takes three steps back to form a larger circle and
  then makes eye contact with others. A head movement is made
  at the same time as eye contact, a nod or slight sideways
  movement, and then the gaze is directed to a point on the wall
  they are facing. Each person moves towards their focus point,
  taking care to negotiate space around other people who may be
  moving in the same or opposite direction.

- Once each person has reached their destination, they turn and
  focus their gaze on a point on the wall furthest away from them.
  Everyone moves briskly to this point, again non-verbally negoti-
  ating space around other people.

- The same format is repeated several times with different forms of
  movement – relevant and within the ranges possible for the
  group.

*Discussion: on different types of energy used in the above exercises. Take this from the
first handshake through to the eye contact with each other and the focus on the point
on the wall, ending with discussion of the type of movement.*

*Main activity (mirror work)*

- In pairs, decide A and B. Person A starts a flowing movement
  using hands. Person B faces and mirrors the movements being
  made. Gradually create more extensive hand and arm movements, then add the shoulders, followed by head, trunk, hip,
  knee and finally foot movements until both A and B are moving
  round the room. Change places so that B leads. Then repeat the
  same format with different types of movement; for example,
  angular, quick and sudden, dainty, clumsy, heavy, graceful
  movements.

- Rest for a while and consider the different types of energy used
  in these exercises. Was there also a particular kind of energy
  created between you and your partner? Discuss this in pairs.

- Stand or sit facing your partner, each person rubbing their hands
  together vigorously with palms inward. Then, hold your hands a

short distance apart, palms facing, and try to feel the energy created by the rubbing movements. Vary the distance between the palms. Repeat this several times; try to imagine a colour that fits the vibrations of energy.

- Repeat this exercise, but hold your hands a short distance from your partner's, so that you feel the energy flow between you. Experiment with distance and create types of energy.

- Discuss the feel of the energies created and the colours that could be associated with them.

- Change partners and find a person who is roughly the same height and build. Stand facing each other. Stand with arms stretched out in front, palms facing your partner's palms. Create a balanced stance for yourself and then move towards your partner so that your palms connect. Make sure you are in a balanced position and then press gently against your partner's palms. Balance may need to be adjusted. The pressure is increased slowly so that each person attempts to unbalance the other.

- Relax and shake hands, arms and legs. Stand back to back with your partner and find different ways of balancing. Then take a few steps away from your partner, remaining back to back. Focus on your balance and imagine a relaxing colour flowing through your body. After a while the colour is concentrated on your spine; imagine the colour flowing up and down your spine, creating a comfortable feeling.

- Move closer to your partner, leaving about 6–12 inches (15–30 cm) space between you, and divide into A and B. Person A imagines their colour flowing through the body. Both people relax and focus on their breathing to become slow, deep and relaxing. Person A now focuses on transmitting the colour from their spine towards their partner. If possible, concentrate for two or three minutes. Relax and then reverse the process so that B transmits colour.

- Discuss in pairs and then the whole group.

*Closure*

- Finish the session by reflecting on the experiences of engaging in the group activity. Say goodbye to the other group members.

*Purpose: to focus on body energies through colour.*

## Session 3

*Warm-up*

- Greet each other and shake hands. Think about the week that has passed and discuss the impact that colours have made upon you. Brainstorm the connections between colour and emotion; for example, red/anger, green/jealousy, yellow/cowardly.

*Main activity*

- The group leader passes round swatches of bright colours. Each person selects one colour. When selection is complete, brainstorm the emotional connections with colours.

- Start to move around the room. Walk briskly and start to loosen up body parts: shoulders, arms, legs, knees, head and neck.

- Now move as if the selected colour is flowing around your body. How does this change the type of movement? Start to move slowly; how does the colour influence slow movement? Start to make larger movements; how does the colour affect the movement?

- Stop and brainstorm on a piece of paper the particular connections you make with this colour. When this is completed, start to cross out words so that only three remain. Decide on the three most important words.

- Move around the room in a manner that conveys the first word; after three minutes or so stop, resume your usual posture and walk around with your usual gait. Move into the second word, allowing about three minutes and then moving into your usual gait and posture again. Then move into the third word. Now walk as if the colour is again moving around your body and allow your body to portray the three words.

- Take another piece of paper and write down the three words and the colour. Consider the words and the way your body felt when you were moving. Decide on the type of person you may have been portraying. Write this type at the head of the paper. Remain with a *type* of person; for example, a busybody, a socialite, a 'hale and hearty' person, an eccentric or a snob.

- When everyone has named a type, resume movement and allow people to embody the type. When the group members have embodied their type, invite them to interact with other types in a non-verbal way.

- Form into two groups standing in a straight line. The line is a bus stop with a timetable on the pole and the bus is due in a couple of minutes. Without words, portray how your character behaves in the queue. Do some feel that being in the queue is beneath them? Are some keen to gain the attention of others? Show your character standing at first: how do you stand? What actions do you make? It becomes obvious that the bus will be late; how does your character react? A lorry goes past and sprays water from a large puddle onto the queue of people. Show how your character reacts. Use any sounds that fit your movements. You see a bus approaching; how does your character react? The bus goes past; it is 'Not in Service'. Show your reaction.

- A car stops and the driver offers a lift. How do you refuse? The bus comes. How do the spaces between people change as it approaches? Relax and shake arms, legs and shoulders.

- Each group shows the other group their short piece of 'work in progress'. Be clear about where the audience should sit or stand.

- After sharing the work shake your body again.

*Closure*

- In a seated circle, reflect on the drama and invite comments on the 'performances' relating to the characters, not as critical comment on performing skills.

- Each person makes a short statement about creating the characters. How did the movements and reactions feel?

- Say goodbye to all the other group members.

*Purpose: to promote awareness of colour and its effect. To start to change usual movements and reactions to others through dramatic media. To begin the process of observing others change their movement patterns.*

## Session 4

*Warm-up*

- Greetings.

- In a standing circle, on-the-spot foot movements as if standing on green, springy grass, then dry yellow grass. Foot and knee movements as if moving through tall green grass; foot, knee and arm movements as if moving through very tall, dry, yellow pampas grass.

- Start to move around the room as if you are moving through a jungle. You need to be careful where you tread and to part vines and branches to move forward. It is very hot. As you reach a safe clearing, stretch and relax.

*Main activity*

- In a standing circle, become aware of your breathing patterns. Start to breathe in and out through your nose. Start to take breath deeper and deeper into your body. Place your hands on your abdomen, palms inwards with your finger tips just touching in the centre of your abdomen just below your navel. Do not press them into your body, just allow them to rest lightly on your clothing. Breathe in gently but deeply and use the breath to part your fingers – they will move back together as you exhale.

- Start to create patterns. Place your arms and hands at your sides and continue with deep breathing. Change the pattern and breathe in through your nose and out through your mouth. Now add a sound to the out breath; start with a soft 'A' – change to a longer sound 'AHAAA'. Create different sounds with vowels and consonants. Stretch and yawn; make the stretch and yawn larger. Create sounds with the yawn. Now make yawn movements with your mouth closed. During this exercise the throat expands; feel this taking place. This is a helpful exercise to perform before speaking as a character or making sounds.

*Soundscape*

- Lie on your back with your head supported by a pillow or small cushion. The group leader reminds everyone of the jungle they moved through earlier. If possible, close your eyes. Start to create some of the sounds that may be present in a jungle: birds, animals, trees, the sounds of the vines parting, the movement of trees. After a while start to listen to other sounds being made as well as your own and begin to respond.

- Suddenly the animals become aware of danger and start to shriek; create these sounds. People have started to use huge electric saws to fell the trees; create these sounds. A tree falls to the ground; create this sound. A huge snake appears and hisses at the people; create this sound. The men run away and the birds are happy; create the bird sounds. Then silence descends.

- Stretch and relax.

- Return to your lying position.

- Relax, close your eyes, allow breath to go deeply into your body and recall your character standing in the bus queue. Allow the colour you chose to flow around your body. As you breathe deeply imagine the colour flowing into your body. How does this feel? Allow the colour to flow around the outside of your body and become aware of the changes to your field of energy.

- As you exhale allow a sound to develop. Relate this sound to your character: what kind of sound might this character make? Is it a high-pitched sound, a low sound or a smooth sound? Start to allow this sound to become louder. At the same time listen to the other sounds that are in the room. Start to interact with the other sounds. Allow the sounds to develop into words – *words* not sentences; for example, some characters may say 'gosh' or 'oh my' or 'hello' or 'sorry'. Try different words and see which fit your character.

- Using these words only, begin to interact with others.

- Relax again and open your eyes.

- Turn on your side and then when you are ready, sit up slowly and then stand.

- Walk slowly around the room and 'recapture' your bus-queue character. Start to say the words created for the character. Do not interact with the others. How do the words inform the way you walk? What kind of rhythm do the words create?

- Stand still and find a gesture that is suggested by the words. This may be large or small. Which parts of your body move? Start to exaggerate the gesture/movement. Start to move around the room making the gesture/movement and sound. Start to interact with others.

- Find a partner and show your gesture and make your sound. Start to interact using only the words, movement/gesture.

- Repeat in groups of three or four.

- Relax and stretch.

- Decide on a particular place for your characters; for example, a pub, a shop, a beach or a waiting room. Devise a short scene. Words can be added but must be informed by the movement/gesture and initial words. Spend a while rehearsing and then each group shows 'work in progress' to other groups.

- Discuss how it felt to take on the persona of the character.

*Closure*

- What would each person like to keep from the character? What would they like to leave behind? Rub off the parts that are to be left behind.

- Say goodbye to the other group members.

*Purpose: to progress to the embodiment phase of character development. To develop character through physicality.*

## Session 5

*Warm-up*

- Greetings.
- Walk around the room, loosening parts of the body that are tense or stiff. Speed up and weave in and out of other people. Now move around other people as though you are being very quiet; signal to other people to be very quiet as well. Now move quickly as if you are in a hurry, signalling to other people to get out of your way. Stand still and look at other people. Now start to move as if you think everyone in the room is less important than you. Then change to demonstrating that you think everyone is more important than yourself. Stand still, move around and release any tension. Move around as if everyone is as important as yourself (and you *are* important).

*Main activity*

- Group leaders should place different one-coloured non-slip mats or similar non-slip materials on the floor.
- Group members move around the spaces between mats (possibly in time to music). In response to a handclap (or when the music stops) everyone stands on a mat (one person per mat) and makes a body shape which represents the energy of the colour. Do not spend time thinking – just respond to the colour. Repeat this several times until people have had the opportunity to experience most or all of the colours.
- Move the mats to one side of the room.
- Walk around the room normally. Group leaders call out the colour of the mats. Each time a colour is called out group members freeze into the shape suggested by the colour, with a period of walking around the room naturally between each 'freeze'.
- Each person selects one shape from the 'freeze' and embodies this shape. Hold the shape in a still position for a while and then start to move around the room, extending the still position into movements.

- Form groups of four or five and create a 'sculpt' or shape from the 'still' positions of the characters. The 'sculpt' will show the relationship between the colour characters.

CREATING A SCULPT

It is very easy to 'do a sculpt' of something. It means taking up a physical stance which expresses what it is you want to say. From this point of view a sculpt is simply a bodily gesture or attitude that stands for, and so gives visible, tangible (sometimes aural) form to a mental idea or attitude. Generally speaking, our bodily gestures are not usually thought out in advance; they occur spontaneously as we find our bodies moving in concert with our minds. Sometimes we have to curb these spontaneous 'sculpts' for fear of expressing things that for one reason or another we want to keep hidden. Bodily gestures and postures are, as everybody knows, extremely revealing because of their tendency to occur spon- taneously, even automatically, showing what we really feel and are thinking at any given moment, whether we choose – or are able – to put it into words or not. We are used to monitoring carefully what our bodies, as well as our facial expressions, are saying, to make sure it is what we want other people to see, so the idea of using our physical presence to 'speak without words' when we actually want to be understood, but find something too painful or too complex or just too awkward to talk about, is obvious. Why not use the way we stand, sit, kneel or lie to make our meaning clear whenever we want to, working out in advance what it is we want to say in this way? The answer is, of course, that verbal commun- ication is, for us, a very powerful cultural constraint, something we need special permission to ignore. Dramatherapy makes a point of granting this permission. It uses sculpts in a wide variety of ways and is always on the look out for new ones. If it can be thought or felt, it can be sculpted.

- Each group shows their 'sculpt' to other group members. This is repeated and the 'audience' is asked to view the 'sculpt' as a family. What are the family dynamics that they see? Who are the family members?
- When each group has heard the suggestions from other group members they remain in the small groups to decide what kind of family they are. Is there a mixture of adults and children? Is this

an extended family? What are the gender, class and cultural issues? What are the relationships between people? Discuss the emotional relationships, remembering that people do not always respond in the same way to emotions that others have for them. For example, an aunt might feel protective towards a niece but the niece may feel resentful of the action this may provoke.

- Each component of the above process should be taken slowly and the leader should ensure that the first stage has been completed before the second stage is suggested.

- End with a sculpt from each group which shows the ages of the family members in a clear way. This will mean some changes in the embodiment but the basic movement will remain the same.

*Closure*

- Walk around the room briskly. Greet other people in the group by name. Shake hands with everyone to say goodbye.

*Purpose: to use colour to start to create more in-depth characters. To start to explore relationships between people. To explore different movement patterns.*

## Session 6

*Warm-up*

- Greetings.

- In a seated circle, start to create different clapping rhythms. Start with a slow beat (maybe to music), then increase the tempo and use different types of rhythm.

- In a standing circle, start to add voice sounds to the clapping rhythms. Vary the clapping by clapping hands against various parts of the body. Change the voice sounds to synchronise with the clapping sounds.

*Main activity*

- Return to the small groups and recap on the family characters. Re-create the sculpts.

- In your own space create the character's body shape. Start to move and as the movement is created begin to focus on the character's rhythm. Create clapping sounds which reflect the movement energy and essence of the character. Add voice sounds. Experiment with different voice sounds until the 'right' sound is found for the character.

- Return to the small groups. Form a seated circle. How will the character sit? Experiment with the kind of gestures your character will make with arms and hands. Begin to make sounds (exclude words) to communicate with others in the circle.

- The occasion is a very happy one. Everyone in the family is pleased. Communicate with hand gestures, sound and facial expression. Repeat this with sad, puzzling, angry and celebratory scenes.

- In the large group, explain to each other how it felt to communicate without words through the characters.

- Return to small groups and in your own space consider the kind of relationship the characters have to one another. Recall the emotional relationships created for the character in session 5.

- Each person has a large sheet of paper and a felt-tipped pen. Create a name for your character and write this at the top of the paper. Underneath write a short character sketch including age, short life history, current environment etc. Do not worry about spelling or punctuation as no one else will be reading your sketch. Allow the pen to write freely.

- In small groups exchange character names and a few key sentences about each character, spoken by the group members as themselves.

*Closure*

- In a large seated circle, say goodbye to your character. Each person speaks for one or two minutes explaining what was liked about your character, what surprises there were (if any), which aspects of the character (movement, voice, characterisation, emotion etc.) could be helpful in your own life and what should be left in the group space.

- Goodbyes.

*Purpose: to develop voice and movement ranges. To develop emotional and communication aspects through a character.*

## Session 7

*Warm-up*

- Greetings.
- Walk around the room as if it is a hot day, then a cold day, then a warm day, then at night, without much light. Move into your character's movement and repeat the above as your character.

*Main activity*

- Move your character through several everyday tasks. (If your character is a child put him or her into a play context.) For example, washing up (perhaps the character does not usually do this and resents the task), eating a sandwich on the move, laying a table or picking flowers. Create the chosen tasks to be in keeping with the kind of character that has been created.

- Form into small groups with chairs arranged in a horseshoe with one chair – the 'hot seat' – in the opening. Each person takes a few minutes to introduce themselves in character to the other group members. The characters then take turns in the 'hot seat' and answer questions. (The questioners are not in character.) The questions should be simple and not too probing. They should help the person in the 'hot seat' to develop the character. Allow about a minute (at least) for the person in the 'hot seat' to form their posture and voice before the others question them for five minutes.

- Return to small groups. Each person repeats the name of their character and others establish what they would call each character – for example, mother, grandmother, Aunt Violet etc. Each person writes the names of all the other characters on a sheet of paper. By or under each name give the emotional response each person elicits from the character of the person who is writing. These should now be more detailed.

*Closure*

- In large circle, say goodbye in character. Each person spends a few minutes on what they could learn from the character.

- Goodbyes.

*Purpose: to develop characters. To explore reactions and responses to others through the character.*

## Session 8

*Warm-up*

- Greetings.

- Walk round the room normally, stretching to release any tension. Find different ways of relaxing and stretching to loosen your body.

- Standing still, make soft sounds. Allow your body to move in response. Make harsher sounds and, again, respond with your body. Make different sounds to move to.

*Main activity*

- Return to small groups. Form a 'sculpt' to find the characters' posture again. Recap on the written work produced in session 7.

- Form into pairs (and one group of three if there are odd numbers). The pairs discuss their emotional responses to each other. Devise a short scene which shows the emotional responses in action. Decide where the scene is set, what it is about, when it is taking place and the particular subject that is being discussed. For example, the place is the kitchen in the home of one of the characters; it is teatime and the subject is the refusal of one of the characters to visit the doctor about persistent headaches. Do not make the scenarios too complicated and do not strain to make them too 'interesting'. Remind people of earlier exercises where people just responded to each other's body movements. Make the scenes like this, except that the responses are to speech and action. Spend a while preparing but do not create a text. For the above example the players may want to decide for how long the headaches have been going on and whether the character usually refuses to visit the doctor.

- Allow 10–15 minutes for rehearsal and then each pair/three shows their piece to other group members. Allow time between each 'performance' for each pair/three to arrange performer/audience spacing. Allow time for feedback and an exploration of, or comments on, the dynamics created in each scenario. This should be observation only, not advice on how it could be improved. Allow time for the actors to de-role before moving on to the next pair/three.

*Closure*

- Discuss the emotions/relationships seen in the performances.
- Goodbyes.

*Purpose: to explore relationships through the dramatic creations.*


## Session 9

*Warm-up*

- Greetings.
- In a standing circle, each person in turn creates a movement. Others copy the movement three times. Repeat, but this time with sound and movement.
- One person stands in the centre of the circle and makes a series of movements. These are repeated three times by the people in the circle.

*Main activity*

- Form into small groups. Devise a scene in which there is a conflict that involves everyone (including children). Decide where the important missing family members are. Their opinions may be important and need to be reported in the scene. Decide where, when and why the family is meeting.

- Rehearse a short scene, allowing 15–20 minutes for the rehearsal. Spend some time on how the audience seating is to be arranged and the effect on the performer/audience relationship.

- Each group 'performs' their scene for the remaining groups. After each scene the actors de-role and listen to feedback about the dynamics the audience has witnessed.

- Following the 'performances' the group discusses the ways the dynamics of the conflict evolved and were dealt with by the characters. How were they different in each group? How did age, class and gender influence the dynamics? Consider the effect of each performance on audience members and actors.

*Closure*

- In a circle, consider what emotions each member wishes to 'leave in the group space' and what considerations people want to take with them.

- Goodbyes.

*Purpose: to explore interpersonal dynamics as actor, audience member and as oneself.*

## Session 10

*Warm-up*

- Greetings.

- Moving around the room to music, each person creates voice sounds for others to move to.

*Main activity*

- Form into small groups. Find a movement for the characters and create a sculpt which shows the conflict. Spend some time devising this sculpt.

- Create a second sculpt showing the conflict resolved.

- Repeat the sculpts. Each group member takes it in turn to step out of the group to view both sculpts. The member is replaced by a group leader if possible. When everyone has done this the group members discuss the comments that were made about their 'performance' in session 9. Do they wish to act on any of these comments? Did they provide helpful insights? The scene is replayed so the ending is as near as possible to the second sculpt.
- Replay the scenes to other group members, starting and ending with the sculpts.
- After each performance the actors de-role and listen to comments from the audience.

*Discussion: how did the characters manage the conflict this time? What were the dynamics?*

*Closure*

- Reflect on how the characters dealt with the conflict. Reflect on the group life and prepare to end the group.

*Purpose: to explore the dynamics of conflict and resolution through drama/theatre as an actor and audience member.*

## Session 11

*Warm-up*

- Find different ways to loosen the body and release tension. Each group member leads a short warm-up.

*Main activity*

- In small groups recapture the characters' movement, voice and energy.
- Repeat 'hot seat' exercises but this time the questions concern how the character contributed to the resolution of the conflict. Were their needs met? How will they get their needs met? How did their inner strength help them?

- De-role and discuss the methods used.
- Say thankyou to each person in the small group. Discuss how each person contributed to the process.
- The whole group discusses the process of the drama.
- Discuss the way that colour can change energies. How did the colours affect the characters' behaviour?

*Closure*

- Say goodbye to the characters. What have people learned from the characters?
- Goodbyes.

*Purpose: to look at how needs can be met during and after conflict. To review how colour can affect body energies.*

## Session 12

*Warm-up*

- Walk around the room, loosening up tension areas of the body.

*Main activity*

- In small groups, create 'sculpts' of the journey through the eleven weeks. Discuss.

*Closure*

- Discuss what people have appreciated about each other.
- Extended goodbyes.

This type of group structure may be helpful for people who are unaware of the dynamics of groups, interpersonal communications and are unable to resolve conflict. This group has focused on conflict but any particular interaction between people could be explored.

The group leader(s) will need to decide how much time is spent on relating the drama to people's own lives.

We now consider some further explorations into role.

## 'Celebrities'

- The group sit in a circle, facing outwards.

    *Leader:* There are lots of people who are famous, but we
    don't know them personally. We see them on TV or
    read about them in the newspapers, or we hear
    people talking about them. As soon as I said 'famous
    people' you probably thought of several people,
    almost all at once. Well, just choose one of them, it
    doesn't matter which. Any one of them will do. I'm
    going to leave a few seconds' pause to give you time
    to decide.

- Group members take it in turns to demonstrate to the rest of the
  group who it is that they have been thinking about. They do
  this silently by pretending to be that person and making a characteristic gesture of theirs or performing an action as they
  imagine that person would do it. The rest try to guess who is
  being imitated. They are allowed only one guess per member.
  Members whose celebrity has been guessed drop out, but the
  rest must stay in the game until they have been identified.
  Because the aim is to be identified, each time their turn comes
  round again they are allowed to vary their action to make it
  more explicit, or to choose a new one (action, not character).
  The winner is the group member whose 'celebrity' is identified
  first.

(To make this easier, group members can be asked to say something in
character as the person they are representing, or easier still, to combine
words and movement.)

## 'Odd one out'

- Group members are given pencil and paper and asked to write
  down a name corresponding to each of the following categories:

  1    Family member (own generation)
  2    Family member (parents' generation)

3   Family member (grandparents' generation)
4   School friend (own sex)
5   Childhood friend or acquaintance (opposite sex)
6   Neighbour
7   Fellow worker or colleague
8   Childhood influence
9   Rival (at school or college)
10  Teacher who influenced me
11  Teacher whom I didn't like
12  Character from novel, play or film (female)
13  Character from novel, play or film (male)
14  TV personality
15  Politician or statesperson
16  Historical character
17  Hero or heroine
18  Person recently in the news
19  An exciting or glamorous job
20  A dull, boring job
21  A job that is difficult to do

- Taking the first three people (1, 2 and 3), ask yourself whether there is a characteristic that two have in common which the other person in the triad lacks. Write the other person's name at the head of a separate list. Then move on to the next triad of names (2, 3 and 4) and repeat the operation. Go on in the same way to the end of the list, recording the 'odd ones out' as you go. It is this list that you will be using in the next step.

- Make up a short story using these people, whether or not you know or have ever met them personally. You need not use the whole list to do this, but at least six of the people in your list must be characters in your story.

- Either tell your story to the other people in the group or write it down and fold the paper up. Folded papers are then jumbled together and placed on a pile in the centre of the circle, for each group member in turn to pick up and read the story written on it to the rest of the group.

## 'Building a character'

*Projection*

- Individuals find their own space.

- Choose someone at random from the list put together in the 'Odd one out' activity. Try not to change your mind once you have decided who to pick.

- Spend some time thinking about this person:

  (a) their history and background, affecting

  (b) their memories, expectations and hopes, governing

  (c) their attitudes to and assumptions about life and the world, influencing

  (d) the kinds of relationship they make with other people and

  (e) the way they tend to behave in particular kinds of circum-stances.

    What are they afraid of, drawn towards, confident about?

    What sort of things do they find it easy to do? Hard to manage?

    What would they be like to go on holiday with? Share a prison cell with? Be told off by?

    Try hard to imagine yourself into the way you think they characteristically feel, think, imagine, react to things.

    What sorts of things have happened to them, and how has it affected them?

    Ask yourself these kinds of questions – but do not take too much time working out the answers. You should have a clear picture of what this person is like – or at least, how she or he *comes over to you*. Ideas will come without you having to make very much effort. Stick with these and move on to the next stage.

- Let yourself think calmly and peacefully about this person. You have been concentrating on writing your list. Now put it to one side and move somewhere else in the room. You can sit down or walk around or lie on the floor (if it is suitable) – whatever is best for thinking about them in a relaxed way, which means thinking *round* them rather than *at* them, and you will find yourself moving gradually into a sense of what it might feel like to be 'in their world'.

- If you are not getting this at all, you are probably trying too hard. Do not give up. Simply think of something else that you like thinking about, and now and again remind yourself of the person you have been concentrating on. How would they fit into it? Do not worry if they would not do. Go on thinking your own thoughts, just keeping in touch from time to time.

- This is the 'visiting' stage of the projection process. Let your mind drift anywhere, and enjoy the freedom to think what you want to. Now and again, drop in on the person you have been thinking about, to see how they are getting on. You need not stay long if you do not want to. Do this three or four times.

- Find someone to share your character with, either by talking about them or demonstrating what they are like.

*Embodiment*

- In your own space again, make a drawing or painting of your character. If you can find things to use you can try making a model of them or a symbol of what you think they are like.

- Try putting yourself in a bodily position ('sculpt') which expresses for you:

    (a)  the way they would stand or lie

    (b)  a pose expressing the sort of attitude you think would be characteristic of them.

- Move about as if you were this person. Standing, walking, running; sitting, lying; picking things up, doing household jobs, arranging things – try your new body out for size. What can you do as this person? What can't you do? What does it *feel* like? Try speaking as this person. What do you sound like to yourself?

- Find a partner and show them. Let them examine your sculpt and observe the way you go about doing things. Speak to your partner in character. Then swap roles with your partner and watch and listen to the character she or he is portraying.

*Role*

- Watch and listen to your partner 'in role' as the character you have created would do this. Reverse roles and repeat.

- Let your partner position you in a sculpt expressing how she or he sees the character you have created. Reverse and repeat.

- In character, let your character meet and introduce him or herself to your partner's character. Then introduce yourselves to another couple. Go on doing this until all the characters have been introduced to one another.

- Still in character, join into groups of three or four and tell the other group members the story of your (character's) life.

- Come out of character in order to put together a dramatic incident involving all the characters in your group. Rehearse this and perform it with the other groups as audience.

- Working on your own again, move round the room 'as yourself'. Try to be conscious of the way your body moves through space, the way your feet hit the ground, the sound of your own breathing etc. Imagine you are somewhere far away from the room you are in – in a meadow, on the beach, walking through a wood, climbing a mountain. These are places you remember and you have been there before – paddling in the streams, running across hot sands, plunging through the undergrowth, gulping in the air.

- Gradually, let the room be itself again. There are people you know, say hello to them and be greeted by them in turn. Are you surprised to see them?

## Working with 'sculpts'

- Working by yourself, try expressing a range of ideas and feelings entirely by means of your bodily posture. To begin with remain in one place, as if you were a statue, then move around the room in this posture. (If you find this impossible take up your sculpt position at various sites in the room.)

- Find a partner and make a sculpt of her or him. You are the 'sculptor' and your partner is the stone, wood, clay etc. which you make into a 'sculpture' simply by moving it (gently) into various positions. Suggested subjects:

  (a)  The way you feel at the moment; or felt when you got out of bed this morning.
  (b)  The way you think people 'see' you.
  (c)  The way you 'see' yourself.
  (d)  The way you 'see' the person you are 'sculpting'.
  (e)  The way you think he/she 'sees' him/herself.
  (f)  The idea or feeling you have about the way things are in your own life-situation, other people's or the world in general.

- After each sculpt you can give your partner permission to move round the room as a 'living statue', or invite other people to come and inspect your work. Then swap roles with your partner so that you are now the 'sculpt' and repeat the process.

- Individuals take turns to make a 'group sculpt' using everyone present or their own selection of people in a group. This is a very powerful way of embodying ideas, attitudes or feelings which represent various strands of the whole. Because several people are involved different feelings may be portrayed in the same sculpt and contrasting themes shown in relationship, either at the same time or in succession. The subject of the sculpt may relate to members' immediate feelings (as when conference dele- gates sum up their impressions of the shared experience they have been passing through during the last hours or days) or it may have a less tangible reference – the use of sculpts to embody abstract ideas (the defeat of oppression and the rebirth of hope or the Spirit of the Nation) or powerful feelings the people share (sorrow, anger, joy, a sense of freedom or injustice); all of these are things that are extremely real – to which the art of sculpting helps to give added impact. (The result resembles the kind of group sculptures often seen in public parks.)

- Because a group sculpt is made of many parts it can be used to portray organisms which hold many things (or people) in tension. The most obvious of these is the human family group. People take turns to build up a group sculpt of their own families, using group members to play the roles needed to form a living family portrait. They may do this completely silently or they can explain why they are choosing particular individuals to play particular parts. As they insert group members into the sculpt they describe to them the people they are representing. This usually turns out to be quite a moving process for the person whose family is being portrayed; so family sculpting needs to be approached with sensitivity and empathy, rather than simply rushed into as 'an interesting thing to do with sculpting'. The emotional impact derives from the fact that sculpting actual personal relationships in this way represents the vital movement from 'embodiment' into 'role'; we are reminded in a powerful way of the reality of our involvement with other people's lives and the way in which our own personal happiness depends on what is *between us and them.*

- This kind of group approach to sculpting may be used to show how individual people have many different characteristics and play a whole range of different roles (what Miller Mair has called 'a conjunction of worlds' (1989, p.250)). Group members take it in turns to choose people from the group to build up a living picture of their own personality, identifying the things they feel are important or revealing about themselves by casting people in roles such as 'my depressed self', 'my musical talent', 'the presence of my mother in my life' etc. This is a very flexible approach.

- Sculpts are a kind of unspoken language and, like all languages, they are most expressive when they communicate by means of contrast. All the above examples of sculpting can be articulated into action processes which demonstrate the movement from one experience into another one which contrasts with it. At its very simplest, if a sculpt can show 'me as I am when I have just woken up', it can also be used to present 'the way I feel when I'm all dressed up for a party'; a group sculpt of the despair of miners' families hearing the news that their menfolk are trapped below ground can change into one showing the reality of their joy when the miners reach the surface again after being released from what seemed certain to be their tomb. Picture flows into picture, so that the possibility of joy is always suggested by the portrayal of grief, because that is how sculpting itself works. The therapeutic use of sculpts depends on this kind of flexibility. Sculpts are never used in a static way but always as part of a process, as unspoken words in sentences where final meaning has not yet been fixed: 'Now let's do it differently …'. Even the kind of group sculpting described above (in which each individual 'casts him or herself' out of the available people so that each person in the group will represent a characteristic to which she or he lays claim) is open to variation, as other people take the opportunity to alter the original sculpt, adding things and changing others: 'What about your kind heart and sympathy for people? You've missed that out!'

# CHAPTER 4

# Self-Disclosure and Disguise

## Dramatherapy and Masks

Dorothy Langley (1983) said that the purpose of masks is always to reveal rather than conceal. We ourselves said something about this in Chapter 3; now we want to take the subject further by looking at what you might call the 'mask-principle' as this applies to drama and to theatre. Concealing in order to reveal, the process whereby we strike at the heart of something by deliberately turning our attention elsewhere, is the essence of theatrical representation. The mask-principle and the theatre principle are the same. It is not only the fact that stage actors traditionally use make-up that is 'made up' about a play. The play itself is fiction, the real lives of the actors concealed behind a mask of make-believe; so why is it that we leave the theatre convinced of its relevance to the truth about our own lives?

It certainly has a lot to do with the way we deal with things that trouble us in our own ordinary lives. Whether we consider ourselves to be strong or weak, cowardly or brave, everybody prefers to avoid being reminded of the things that disturb or trouble us about life in general and their own lives in particular. It is a psychological fact that anything that frightens, alarms or appals us about the future, makes life difficult and burdensome in the present, or reminds us consciously or unconsciously of sufferings endured in the past and still exerting their power over us today, is kept at a distance by us, and that we do this automatically – so automatically in fact that we usually do not know we are doing it. In order to take away the power of these fears to affect our lives in ways we cannot control and do not understand, and to heal these wounds, they must somehow be recognised and understood, and their power to disturb us acknowledged. This is a process we resist because it is painful – sometimes very painful indeed. This, of course, is the main argument behind psychoanalysis. Freud himself stated that 'The task of the therapist lies in overcoming...

this resistance to association' (Freud 1895, p.87) and warned his patients that they 'must never lose sight of the fact that a treatment like ours proceeds to the accompaniment of a constant resistance' (Freud 1909, p.229).

Somehow, theatre manages to get under our guard and remind us in no uncertain terms of the things we are avoiding, or at least trying so very hard to avoid. Because it is a projective approach, and directs attention away from our own personal lives towards a fictional scenario which, however much it resembles the state of affairs we may be involved in, exists on a different plane altogether in 'a world of its own', theatre avoids the defences we put up. The paradox is that it does this by assuring us that we do not really need to take it all that seriously. Even the most serious, even tragic, play comes across to part of our mind, the consciously censoring part, as a game, a particularly ingenious kind of trick. After all, it is just made up, isn't it? A product of someone's imagination. What we overlook when we dismiss theatre in this way is that any play which we enjoy or appreciate is a function of *our own* imagining as well as that of the author, actors, designers and director. At the level of imagination there is no argument, no agreement to differ, but all is genuinely shared. This is the way that imagination penetrated to the source of our emotional problems, working behind the back of our ability to judge what is 'real' or not. A play is a theatrical mask which reveals the truth to us – which is why in the sixteenth and seventeenth centuries allegorical dramas, plays with 'hidden' meanings, were called 'masks'.

Because it works in this contradictory or paradoxical way, being both true and false, real and fantasised at the same time, drama specialises in things which seem to run counter to each other and yet be mutually dependent. It is the ideal format for those aspects of human experience which pull us in two directions at once:

- the urge to reveal ourselves and the contradictory urge to remain safely hidden from view

- the need to be individual and at the same time belong to the crowd

- the desire to remain open to other people while preserving one's defences against them

- the longing to 'live dangerously' in complete safety

- the urge to extend one's horizons without having to venture into unknown territory.

All these, and others one could think of, are actually variations on the same theme of safety and danger. The summons to embrace being human, being alive, is always a call to take on things which may go disastrously wrong or involve oneself in situations which will obviously involve personal suffering of some kind or another. Landy (1993), in his study of dramatic role, uses the idea of *role-distance* to explain the way in which taking on a part in a play – assuming the 'mask of drama' – allows us to behave more courageously than we would normally do. The fact that the role I am playing in the drama obviously is not really me at all gives me the freedom ('distance') to express my feelings, attitudes and desires in an undercover way. If I am *this* (the personage in the play) I cannot be accused of being *that* (the vulnerable person I feel myself to be). Thus the roles we take on in plays act like masks, encouraging us to take risks with ourselves; and this is true whether or not the play is actually being presented in a theatre.

This kind of role-distance gives us a clue to the way that plays themselves are like masks, allowing a kind of trade-off between safety and danger, so that we can take risks and yet remain protected by the fact that it is after all only a play. To understand this properly, however, we need to look at the concept of *catharsis* as well as role-distance, and see how the two things belong together. Catharsis means 'being purged by emotion'. It is the oldest theory of how theatre and drama work (in the western world at least) and was first put forward by Aristotle (*Poetics*, vi, 2). Being so ancient does not make it any less relevant to modern theatre, however. The principle of creating a healing effect through the release of emotional tension has been used by generations of psycho-spiritual therapists since – and probably before – Aristotle spelled it out for us. He sees it happening specifically within a theatrical setting, but it can be reproduced in other places too. Catharsis takes place wherever the degree of emotional threat can be answered by and balanced with the level of psychological safety.

Drama sets reality at a distance, so that to be in a play is, in itself, a relatively *safe* occupation, so long as nobody else is watching; nobody outside the play, that is. But when people *are* watching, when there is an audience, it becomes theatre and then the stakes are much higher as the risk of exposure is so much the greater. At the same time, of course, the possibility of acceptance has also increased. Drama offers us an alternative world, a world of imagination that is both safe – being imaginary – and exciting, because of the opportunity it gives us for self-expression. Thus a play allows us to be ourselves by pretending to be someone else; this is the paradox of drama.

In fact, it is not really a paradox. Drama and theatre function within the sphere of the imagination, and imagination is the faculty we use in order to make things real for ourselves. Their basic task is to set reality – current reality, the one we are used to – at a distance, and to offer us an alternative one which we may either accept or reject. If we choose to accept it then we possess the ability, the imaginary power, *to make it real for us*. The process is clearly demonstrated in theatre, where the 'world' of the play, the imaginative alternative reality, is separated from the 'ordinary' world of the audience by an actual physical space. From this point of view theatres are places where people stand in queues and pay money (unless they are lucky enough to have complimentary tickets) to watch other people risk revealing these innermost feelings and thoughts so that they, the audience, can open themselves up to feeling in touch with life at less emotional expense. Because they know it is a play and they are only the audience, they feel safe enough to join in; because it is a play about human beings – men, women and children like themselves – they are drawn across the space that divides and protects, and involved in the action.

A well-known version of Aristotle's teaching is Sue Jennings' (1990) 'ritual-risk paradigm':

> The ritual factor creates the safety, the predictable, the known. It may be the map we look at before we start a journey. It may be the movement, chants or song that the group creates to start and end; it is a statement which acts as a container for change, for the journey, for the adventure. The risk factor is the unexpected, it catches us unawares, it is the unknown journey and can take us into uncharted territory. (Jennings 1990, p.62)

This is catharsis in operational terms, as it takes place in dramatherapy designed as a special vehicle for mediating the confrontation between safety and danger. The unexpected, unknown element stands in fact for things that are really well known – much too well known, in fact. When Jennings describes 'the adventure' dramatherapy presents, she is talking about the way that we are led by the drama into areas of life which are 'unknown', 'unexpected', 'frightening', because they represent the kind of knowledge borne of personal experience that we ourselves have made strange, unknown, other, by refusing to allow ourselves to recognise its existence: the terrors and despairs we have known and lived through and deliberately 'forgotten', but whose wounds we still bear in our lives. Dramatherapy, like other kinds of dynamic psychotherapy, aims at giving these wounds an opportunity to begin to heal, by making them an acknowledged part of our 'journey' towards wholeness – bringing them out into the open, in fact.

Writing about the way that catharsis originates in early childhood experience, Thomas Scheff (1979) describes how 'the child draws into himself [sic] to feel the pain, puts his head down and cries, but frequently looks at his mother to see if the situation is still safe. While feeling the pain, the child also sees himself through the mother's eyes' (Scheff 1979, p.62). In other words, the suffering individual, in this case the child, achieves a degree of distance from their suffering by taking on the role of someone else; this is not done in order to deny the pain, but to gain some kind of help in living through the pain. The distance between child and mother – the fact that they are two separate people – allows the child to draw on someone else's love in order to gain courage to endure what is happening. In other words, the child's ability to bear pain is reinforced by relationship, by the distance between two people who are able to turn to each other in love.

It is important to understand that it is the distance which separates and defines their identity that allows them to do this. At such times, in order to bear being themselves, people need real help from elsewhere, even if it is only permission to weep. In fact, the mother's reaction to her child's pain helps to establish the reality and acceptability of the pain for the child. According to Scheff, being allowed to cry helps children adjust to the burdens which 'appear to be an inescapable feature of infancy as a result of intense and incommunicable feelings of separation and loss' (1979, p.62). And this, of course, is what plays do. They give us permission to weep. Within this shared world of imagination, made real for us by the factual presence of other real people, we find courage to be ourselves. Because we are supported and reinforced by this ability to share other people's feelings by identifying them with our own, we are able to break through into accepting the things we have not really let ourselves feel before and have always managed to keep at a distance.

That distance was unacknowledged, however. We pretended that it was not there and that we were accepting everything, feeling all there was for us to feel. Drama is designed to bring the distance home to us. We look across at other people's pain and because it belongs *to them as well as to us* we allow ourselves to acknowledge feelings which at other times and in other places we have succeeded in avoiding having to take on board. Distance and safety go together; the more distanced we are from our real awareness of the presence of whatever it may be that terrifies us about ourselves and other people, the safer we begin to feel. Sharing our imagination provides a safe way of meeting other people and this turns out to be a way in which we can also make contact with ourselves, too. Drama represents a distanced encounter with feelings and ideas that need to be incorporated in the way that we consciously express ourselves. It is a way of letting ourselves be unmasked.

This balance between safety and danger, which allows us to find a way of accepting the presence of our own pain, is the secret of catharsis. Scheff (1979) describes how people who are protected and exposed at the same time can abandon their psychological defences and begin to face aspects of reality they have trained themselves to deny. Situations favourable to catharsis are simply ones in which we feel secure enough to 'see ourselves feeling' – to face the fact that we are actually moved and upset. This happens most strikingly in theatres, where we are quite literally and obviously separated from whatever is going on on-stage, and because of this we feel free to leap the gap and allow ourselves to become imaginatively involved with what is going on in front of us so that we really feel ourselves to be part of that world, vividly aware of the experience of sharing its life. At the same time we remain fully aware that this in fact is not our world and we are safe from the things that are happening in it, because drama allows us the privilege of 'identification without assimilation' – although we identify with the people in the play, we do it in a way that acknowledges their otherness and avoids trying to make them part of ourselves.

This 'keeping at a distance' is what makes drama work as a healing experience. As such, it lies at the very heart of dramatherapy. In drama and in dramatherapy there is no confusion between the reality I am afraid of and the safe one I have privately constructed in order to hide myself from the private, secret fears. This is an altogether different kind of image-building, where the element of make-believe is quite explicit; we find ourselves playing creatively with other people and enjoying the game. This important difference between private fantasy and shared imagination is where drama and theatre start from, and it gives them the ability to speak on behalf of every kind of distance within and between people that cries out to be taken up into relationship and healed. So long as dramatherapy is able to find ways of getting people to create this kind of imaginative sharing it will be both fully dramatic and authentically therapeutic. As Peter Brook says, 'The actor does not hesitate to show himself exactly as he is, for he realises that the secret of his role demands his opening himself up, disclosing his own secrets' (Brook 1968, p.60). People taking part in a dramatherapy session are all actors from this point of view, people who are willing to use role in this way, as a means of achieving honesty about themselves. The purpose of dramatherapy structures and processes is to enable them to feel confident to let go of their disguises, at least temporarily, so that in time they may become less attached to them. Dramatherapy is about abandoning this kind of mask.

To summarise, then. In the language of mask we drop one kind in order to take up another, as the psychological mask is abandoned in favour of the dramatic, the purpose of which is not to disguise but to reveal. As Jennings says, 'Masks can contain the feelings that could not otherwise be expressed' (1990, p.116). Walter Sorrell (1973) points out that some of these feelings may not be acceptable to anyone at all, being socially proscribed as well as simply painful to the person who has them and suffers from them. Looking at masks from an anthropological point of view, he is able to add another to the list of contrasting feelings expressed in or embodied by masks: religious and social rituals throughout the world reveal the fact that humankind has a 'need for self-repulsion as well as total possession of himself' (Sorrell 1973, p.7). There is an unacceptable side to life itself, to *simply being human*, which emerges in masked rituals in order to do battle with whatever is good, true and loving in individuals, communities and the human race itself. The purpose of the ritual, of course, is to allow the tables to be turned so that good can be seen to triumph mightily over evil. In this way, the rite serves the purpose of distancing the performers from evil, demonic forces inside themselves or at loose within society as a whole.

The psychologist C.G. Jung pointed out that, in classical Greek theatre, the use of masks was understood to fulfil two very important purposes, which are connected but not identical. First, there was the cathartic purpose – that of providing protection for the wearer's vulnerability while at the same time allowing them to express their own individuality (the Greek word for mask, *persona*, actually means 'something sounded through', because the actor's own voice sounds through the mask). Second, and equally important, was the archetypal identity of being portrayed by the actual mask itself, which 'symbolised the unification of the individual ego with the hidden ancestors dwelling in him ... For him who wears the mask, all taboos are abolished' (Jacobi 1976, p.37). As we have said, the experience is one of both *protection* and *liberation*, as 'the collective background moved into the foreground, bestowing on those identified with the archetypal level both freedom and security' (Jacobi 1976, p.38).

All this seems a long way from an ordinary dramatherapy session, although dramatherapy is never ordinary in the sense of being dull and lacking in interest. Any group that decides to experiment with masks should be prepared for the possibility that ideas of this sort will certainly come to the surface. The quietest, most subdued people, given the chance to make a mask for themselves, produce images of demons. 'Image' is the wrong word, however; what begins with a pictorial image becomes a terrifying and demanding presence, as the person we knew, whose gentleness and restraint we appreciated so much, is instantly transformed before us, simply by putting on a home-made mask. The impression is irresistible that this is not a mask but a living creature; so long as the mask stays on, the impression stays too, and nothing really succeeds in persuading us to the contrary.

The simple fact is that people take on the characteristics of the mask they are wearing. In anthropological terms 'Masks tame spirits by claiming their powers' (Sorrell 1973, p.8); tame them and also enlist them, as we begin to discover things about themselves, their own potentialities and powers that they never imagined. To don a mask can be a very strange experience indeed, and sometimes an exceedingly surprising one, as you discover that these strange, even bizarre, features were in fact 'made' for you – whether this is literally true or not.

The subject of masks and the subtitle of this book go together in the most striking way. In the Greek myth of Perseus and Andromeda, no one could rescue Andromeda from the terrifying Gorgon, Medusa, whose glance alone was enough to turn people into stone. The hero Perseus, however, held his shield in front of himself as he reached across to rescue her. The Gorgon saw her own face reflected in the burnished shield and was destroyed by the image. Thus, Perseus mastered his terrors by reflecting them back upon their source.

Something needs to be said at this point about the need for boundaries. The immediate effect of having one's current and habitual role blown wide open in this way can be overpowering. Some people may need active encouragement to enjoy 'being' this new creature; others have to be reassured that they are in fact still themselves and in control of their own reactions. Most of us need a little of both. Sometimes it is necessary to restrain somebody who seems about to go over the top and get carried away. It is easy to take masks off but their effects tend to last longer than you would expect. That, however, is the whole point; that is why they have a lasting effect in therapy, serving to remind us of a time when we discovered powers we never knew we possessed, an experience we can relive in our imagination way into the future.

Sue Jennings' book *Dramatherapy with Families, Groups and Individuals: Waiting in the Wings* (1990) has a chapter on 'Masks and unmasking' which is highly recommended. In it she describes and demonstrates the use of characters and situations drawn from mythology as an effective way of creating dramatic distance: 'The way of the mask is rich and infinite, and brings together both an art form in itself and a therapeutic journey for therapist and client alike' (Jennings 1990, p.128).

To sum up, masks give us courage to take part in drama, and to lose ourselves in dramas which are on things that happen to other people, by allowing us to express what would otherwise stay hidden, both from others and from ourselves. We may need to hold on to some of the things we liberate in ourselves and not just flush them away. We may need to find ways of embodying our demons, so that our catharsis may really become empowerment.

The following example of group work with masks has a 12-week group structure.

**Session 1**

- Standing in a circle, introduce yourselves to one another (see 'Group rules and group culture', p.59).

- One by one, start to move your shoulders up and down. Pass this movement round the group.

- In sequence, start to move your feet, knees, hips etc. so that each part of your body is flexed and relaxed.

- Take it in turns to occupy the centre of the circle. Move your whole body so that the others can imitate your action.

- Next, cover one hand with the other one, palm to palm. Make a rocking movement with your two hands, without separating them. Still holding your hands together, try out different relationships between your hands, your arms, your body. How many ways can you move one hand against the other without your hands losing contact with each other (e.g. washing, rubbing, striking, pushing etc.)?

- Come out of the circle and walk round the room using your hands to touch different surfaces or textures. Choose one or two surfaces which you find interesting. Take someone else to see or feel these.

- What are these surfaces covering or masking (e.g. paint on a wooden surface, wallpaper on a wall etc.)?

- Share your ideas and feelings about what you have been doing. What does it tell you about the way we use one thing to cover, protect, decorate or draw attention to something else?

**Session 2**

- Greetings. Stand in a circle. Breathe deeply, stretching upwards and outwards, then relax and flop as you expel all the air, before drawing air in and stretching again.

- This time, yawn as you expel the air. Repeat this several times. Stretch and yawn at the same time. Keeping your face in the yawning position, stand with your hands by your sides.

- Put your hands in front of the lower half of your face to hide it from view; then change the expression of your mouth behind your hands. Try this several times. Then keep one of the expressions you have been trying out and show it to the group without hiding it with your hands; and then just relax.

- Find another expression behind your hands. How would someone wearing this expression move hands, shoulders and other parts of their body? Stay where you are and experiment.

- In pairs, show your expression to your partner. Ask them to reproduce it back to you. Show them how to move their bodies in line with that expression. Then let your partner show you their expression and the movements that go with it.

- Help your partner to experiment by fitting expressions to movements. Move round the room doing this, before changing places and moving round again.

*Discussion: how did it feel to take on a particular expression and the movements that went with it? How did it feel to have someone else take on your expression and movements? Talk this over, sharing your ideas and feelings.*

## Session 3

- Greetings. Stand in a circle. Warm up by shaking different parts of your body etc.

- Position your hands on different parts of your body, then move your body towards your hands. Shake your hands loosely.

- Put your hands a few inches away from your mouth to hide it, then communicate with other people using only your eyes so that they cannot see the expression revealed by your mouth. This is done by putting your mouth into a particular expression behind your hand, and then conveying it to the others by what they see in your eyes. Go on to try different expressions.

- Sitting down, draw or paint a mouth on the front of your hand (which is still covering your *real* mouth). Give this painted mouth a particular expression.

- Draw another mouth with a different expression on the sole of your shoe, one that really shows how you feel. You now have two painted-on mouths, the one by your real mouth 'saying' one thing, the other on your shoe communicating the opposite feeling.

- Talk from behind your hand, revealing as much or as little about how you really feel as you want or feel able to do. While you are doing this you can show the drawing on your shoe as much or as little as you want.

*Discussion: what have the group been doing? How did it make them feel?*

- Pairs stand back to back, one partner expressing the feeling that both want to present to the world, while the other expresses their actual feelings. They act as one person, communicating their feelings by bodily posture and facial expression.

- Pairs form a two-person sculpt expressing how they would like things to be for each of them.

## Session 4

- Greetings. Stand in a circle. Warm up. Spend a little time concentrating on facial expressions.

- Pass a pair of spectacles (minus lenses) around the group, each person trying them on and telling the others what it feels like to do this. Do the same thing with a funny hat and then a red nose.

- Choose a pair of specs, hat or nose. Look in the mirror. What kinds of movements are suggested by these things? Experiment with wearing them, adding other things until you have built up a kind of half-mask, checking out how you look in the mirror as you go along.

- Give your mask a name.

- Create an environment for your mask and discover the ways that it would move around in its environment.

- Invite other masks in to build up a shared environment with you and interact using movement before paying a joint visit in which half the group receive the other half as guests.

- Take off your masks and de-role. Reflect on the drama created before saying goodbye to one another.

## Session 5

- Greetings. Move around the group space warming up the body: feet, knees, legs, hips, shoulders, arms, hands, trunk, neck and head.

- Become aware of the parts that are the most difficult to warm up – the parts of the body that hold the most tension. Spend more time on these areas. Stroke them, massage them, maybe ask someone else to massage them for you.

- Allow yourself to become aware of the part of your body which relaxes most readily, which part of your body feels most comfortable. (It may take a while to bring this body part to mind as we are usually most aware of areas that bring discomfort.)

- As a whole group, use the space you have to map out the area of a body. Decide at which end of the room the head will be, where the trunk will be and the position of the feet. Mark these places with chairs.

- Within this framework, move to the area corresponding to the part of you that relaxes most easily. For example, if your knees always feel flexible and comfortable, stand in the space designated for knees. Adopt a comfortable standing position. Allow breath to flow deeply and evenly through your body.

*Create the* feeling *of this part of your body rather than trying to* become *this part of your body. Stretch and feel the calmness flowing through the whole of your body.*

- Now use facial expressions, arms, hands, any part of your body in order to make contact with other people without leaving your chosen place.

- When facial contact has been made, start to move towards other people, maintaining calm and relaxed movements.

*Discussion: what kinds of unifying movements can be made with other people?*

- Devise a group scenario to show the unification of the relaxed body parts within the body-shape the group has made.

- Now leave the body-shape and move into individual spaces. Consider the links between the facial expressions and the body. Draw an image of the face and body in which the calmness felt in the selected body part is illustrated in the face. Using blank ready-made masks create the mask of the body part.

*Equipment: you will need a selection of paints, felt-tipped pens, crayons, coloured tissue paper, fabrics and assorted items that may be used to decorate the mask. Also staplers, glues, scissors and pastes.*

- Complete the session by sharing the completed masks. Put masks into boxes. Say goodbye to each other calmly.

## Session 6

- Greetings. Collect masks. Each person spends a while looking at his or her mask and 're-connecting' with it.

- Put the masks on a ledge or table so they can 'view' their creators. Begin to go through the movements you tried out in session 5.

- Hold your mask in one hand and incorporate it into your move-ments. Repeat the movements several times.

- Place the mask over your face and secure it to your head; then look at yourself in a mirror (full length if possible). Re-create the movements and explore the effect of wearing the mask. (If this feels uncomfortable at any point remove the mask and replace it on the ledge or table where it can 'view' you again.)

- Wear your mask to move around the room connecting with the other masks. Start to make some quiet sounds. When it feels appropriate slowly increase the volume. Show the mask charac-ters miming everyday actions: eating, drinking, catching a bus, driving a car. Remove masks and place them in their viewing positions. Shake and stretch as needed. Reflect verbally on the whole experience of wearing the masks.

- Recall the part of your body that was the most tense. Become aware of the kind of movement that this tension creates in your whole body.

- Repeat the body exercise in session 5 but this time focus on the body part that holds the most tension.

- Now stand in front of your 'calm' mask and re-create the movements connected with this mask. Then spend some time adjusting these movements so all the tension you have been creating in yourself is dissolved.

- As a group, reflect on the drama created in the session. Rub your body with your hands to rid yourself of any uncomfortable feelings, then shake these feelings from your hands. Put masks into boxes.

- Say goodbye to one another.

## Session 7

- Greetings. Walk around the room warming up your body. Take your mask from the box and place it in the 'viewing' position.

- Begin to change your movements into those you associated with tension. Go on to create a mental and physical image of the facial expression connected with the tense body.

- Make a second mask representing this state. (You will need the same kinds of materials.)

- Now incorporate the new mask into the movement. Put it onto your face and look at yourself in a mirror. Re-create the movements that go with the mask. How are these affected by wearing the mask?

- Remove mask and place the two masks side by side.

- Now put a large sheet of paper next to each mask. Brainstorm words connected with the mask and write them down on the appropriate piece of paper. (Aim for at least six words on each piece.)

- Write a short character sketch for each mask, incorporating the words already on the two sheets of paper. Name each mask.

- To close the group, introduce your two masks to other group members.

- Put masks into boxes. As you put your own masks into the box say what you are putting in along with them:

  *For example, 'I am putting my tension mask whose name is [insert name] into the box. With him/her I am putting the physical and emotional pain that I associate with him/her.'*

- When everyone has put everything they need to into the boxes (actually and symbolically) then move on to say goodbye.

## Session 8

- Greetings. Collect masks. Move around the room to warm up.

- Take your masks from the box and put on your first mask, the calm, comfortable one. Now move around the room as this mask.

- Put this mask into the 'viewing' position and replace it with your second mask. Move around the room wearing this mask.

- Remove this mask and place it in a position that allows the first mask (the calm, comfortable one) to view the second mask. The first mask must be in the dominant position.

- Arrange the chairs so that you are sitting in the shape of a horseshoe, with one chair positioned in the gap, facing the horseshoe. This is the 'hot seat'. Take it in turns to sit in this seat, wearing your first mask. (Find the right physical position in the chair to fit your mask.)

- Reply to questions put to your mask by the people sitting in the horseshoe. These should be simple ones (e.g. 'Do you like flowers?', 'Which is your favourite season and why do you like it?' etc.) rather than questions designed to delve into the psyche. This can go on for about three minutes, then allow time for each person to de-role before the next person sits in the chair. Return the masks to their original positions after they have been worn.

- Put on your first mask. *As the mask character*, take up a typical posture and say what you have learnt about the other mask.

- Form a group picture or sculpt wearing the masks (as if a group photograph were to be taken).

- Place the masks into the boxes, repeating the same closure as for session 7.

- Say goodbyes.

## Session 9

*Remind group of number of sessions left.*

- Greetings. Warm yourselves up.

- Take your masks from the boxes and re-connect with them.

- Place the first (calm, comfortable) mask in the viewing position and wear the second mask. Now re-create the movements for the second mask.

- Find a partner whose movements are more or less similar to yours. Begin to interact with your partner through the medium of movement.

- Remove your mask and reflect on the movements you have just created. With these movements as your stimulus, devise a short scene together. Replace masks and improvise the scene with each other.

- Show your improvised scene to the other group members.

*First spend a few moments deciding where the audience of other group members will sit, so that the sharing now becomes a piece of theatre. Make sure that the 'viewing' masks can still view! Also allow time for performers to de-role before moving on to the next performance.*

- Reflect on these scenes and the way they were performed from both perspectives – audience and performers.

- Put masks into boxes in the way that you did in session 8.

- Say goodbyes.

## Session 10

- Greetings. Warm up.

- Remove masks from boxes. Mask 2 is placed in a viewing position. This should not be in the same place as formerly occupied by Mask 1 in the previous session.

- Put on your mask; remember and re-create your movements, act a short scene in which the masks discuss the performances they viewed in session 9. Remove your masks and reflect, in pairs then in the whole group, on the discussion between the masks.

- Replace your masks and create another scene in which the masks show how Mask 1's influence on Mask 2 could be more powerful.

- Share these scenes with the group.

- Reflect on the performances, sharing ideas and feelings as in session 9.

- Replace masks in boxes. Say goodbyes.

## Session 11

*Remind group that this is the penultimate session.*

- Greetings. Body warm-up. Take masks from boxes.

- Put Mask 1 in the 'viewing' position. Put on Mask 2 and walk around the room acknowledging the other masks.

- Discuss the performances you watched and presented in session 10 (a) in pairs; (b) as a whole group.

- Create a short performance entitled 'How [names of the two second masks] used the wisdom of [names of the two first masks]'.

- Show the performance to the rest of the group.

- Reflect on the performances.

- Put your masks back in the box. Say goodbyes (these can be quite extended).

## Session 12

- Greetings. Take masks from the boxes.
- Reflect together on the ways that the masks have influenced body, mind and spirit.
- Decide what you each want to do with your masks.
- To consolidate your experience within the group, make each person in the group (including yourself) a personal picture-card, showing the mask you would like them to wear (i.e. the way you would like them to present themselves).
- Distribute the cards and say goodbye to everyone, taking some time to do this properly.

*Groups should be followed up:*

- *to discover their impact on people's day-to-day lives*
- *to reflect on the future progress of people in the group*
- *to complete the process of group dispersal and closure.*

The following case study involved individual therapy with masks in multiple one-hour sessions.

## Debra: A case study

Debra is 23. She has a history of self-harm since the age of 12, mostly cutting arms and legs, inducing infection after body piercing and tattoos. Her father left the family home when she was 6 and has had no further contact with her, her mother or her two sisters. She felt lonely and isolated during childhood and was bullied at infant, junior and secondary schools. Debra described her mother as loving and caring; she worked hard to support the family after the father left. Debra did not tell her mother about the bullying at school.

Her current social situation is that she has lived with a male partner for two years. She feels secure in this relationship but not ready to commit herself to marriage, although he would like to formalise the partnership. Her mother lives in the same town. Debra describes her relationship with her mother and her siblings as 'distant'. Debra works as a florist. She enjoys her work, but would like to own her own shop.

She is unable to pinpoint any specific life events that prompted her self-harming behaviour. She cannot recall the first time she cut her arms and legs with a razor. This was always a secret action and she wears thick tights or socks and long sleeves to avoid scars being seen. She had always feared she would be exposed at school, thus she avoided sports or activities when she would need to wear short sleeves. She was often scolded by teachers and teased by peers for wearing long sleeves but 'enjoyed' having a secret. She has always enjoyed watching the released blood flow away from the wound and the feeling of 'relief and release' of the actual opening of the skin. She feels ashamed and silly after the event. Tattoos and body piercing have 'greater pain' for her but not to the same level of fascination. The introduction of infection provides an opportunity to talk to other people. Debra would like someone to challenge her about the infections but no one has ever verbalised the suspicions that she believes people do harbour. Debra describes cutting as an addiction. She enjoys the element of secrecy but would like to be found out.

Debra says she feels 'detached' from her body. Seeing the blood flow from the wounds reminds her that she is alive. Later, she has a sense of self-disgust and loathing. Debra has chronic feelings of low esteem. She has no sense of self-worth.

She says she has come to therapy because she would like to increase her self-esteem and find a degree of self-worth. She wants to stop her self-harming behaviour and put an end to the resulting feelings of shame and guilt.

The initial sessions were spent on history taking and exploring the sensations Debra experiences when she is engaging in self-harm.

*Session 1*

The history of blood-letting as a medical practice was introduced by the therapist. No comments or direct links were made with her current situation but Debra did do some research on her own and at the next session she commented that all the illustrations she had found were of male doctors performing the blood-letting. Again, no analysis was made in relation to this statement.

*THERAPIST'S THOUGHTS AND REFLECTIONS*

*To engage Debra in therapy we need to explore the secret elements of her behaviour and the importance of what having a secret means to her. The therapy should enable her to 'connect' with her body in a creative manner. The images that are strongest are the flowing blood and the scars that remain to remind her of her actions.*

### Session 2

During the session the therapist

- explores with Debra the differences between male and female healing. Debra is unsure about this division but is sure that she dislikes the images of males that she has been looking at. She starts to discuss female healing which she sees as gentle and caring. She links this with the aspect of cutting that she enjoys most, the flowing of the blood and the symbolism of the blood as a life force.

- discusses Debra's work as a florist and how she engages with her creative impulses within the constraints of the level of work she is permitted to do. She enjoys the colours of the flowers and the displays she can create with them. She particularly enjoys making bridal bouquets because of the colour and textures of the flowers. This is the only creative outlet she has at present.

- explores Debra's views of the opposite of 'flowing' (a positive word/concept for her). She thinks for about three or four minutes and offers the words 'stuck', 'fixed' and 'blocked'.

No interpretations or comments are made by the therapist. Although the therapist has already discussed the indirect nature of dramatherapy with her, this is returned to as an area of discussion and as a basis for the therapy contract.

*THERAPIST'S THOUGHTS AND REFLECTIONS*

*The creative work that is familiar to her, colour and texture, should be the starting point for the creative focus of the therapy. The opposites of male/female, stuck / flowing and the connections she had made with these should influence the art form. As she is disconnected from her body the embodiment phase should follow projective work because focusing on her body too soon could induce increased self-harm both for comfort and also as a method of checking she exists. Mask work is to be considered because masks will link with her current creative expression because of the kind of craft involved; they will form a projective option which will initially focus on the face before moving to embody the mask characters; the images she has presented will form the basis for the mask work and will suggest a structured approach.*

### Session 3

During the session the therapist discusses this proposed plan of action with Debra, who says she understands and agrees with it. Various methods of making masks are discussed. Debra says that she prefers the method of using plaster of Paris bandage to create the masks from her own face. She feels it is important 'to create from her own image' (a phrase that is noted by the therapist and will be introduced at a later stage). Using this method will involve touch by the therapist. Debra agrees to the physical contact and also understands that some preparation will be necessary. This preparation includes her becoming familiar with the contours of her face. She applies face creams twice a day, performing these actions slowly and sometimes without looking in the mirror in order to heighten the sensation of touch. (This is also a useful start to the later stages of therapy when gentle contact with her body can be introduced in order to replace cutting.)

During the session the therapist engages Debra in some exercises which involve the therapist touching her head, face and shoulders. These include gentle massaging, attaching hair accessories and discovering the positions in which Debra feels most comfortable about having her face touched. Following this, thin veils and scarves are used to cover all or part of her face. She is encouraged to view the transformations in a mirror. When these warm-ups have been completed and she feels comfortable with touch and having her face covered, two masks are made. This process involves covering her face with a lubricant and adding layers of tissue paper before applying the plaster of Paris bandage. (This did not cover her nostrils, mouth or eyes.) As plaster of Paris dries very quickly the masks are hardened by the next session.

Debra decides that the masks will represent these two aspects:

- Mask 1 – Female, wise, healing, flowing.
- Mask 2 – Male, harsh, stuck, barren, bullying.

The healing mask is decorated first. This work is undertaken during three sessions and is carried out with intense concentration on Debra's part. She uses paints, felt-tipped pens, silk flowers and leaves, glitter glue, embroidery silks and wool to create a mask of a young woman who wears a serene expression and has flowers entwined in her long black hair. The result is a stylised rather than naturalistic representation of a face. The mask has a motif of painted flowers outlined with glitter on the forehead. The lips are created from red tissue paper. When the mask is complete Debra expresses some surprise about her ability to create an artefact of such beauty from the contours of her own face.

The second mask is very different. Debra starts by making a black mark on the forehead with a thick felt-tipped pen. She states that this represents 'badness oozing out' but does not make any further comment. After staring at the mark for some time she eventually mixes some dark red powdered paint into a thick paste and, with a thick paint brush, applies some of this colour to the edges of the eye-holes. Next she says she wants to look at the mask from a distance to gauge the effect that the colours have made on the white base. She is uncertain about how to proceed, saying she has no clear image of how she wants the completed mask to appear. She agrees to allow the paint to dry before she proceeds on to the next session. She states that she does not find the mask frightening but that it does not seem 'to be suggesting ways to go with it' in the way that the first mask had. (When working with masks people often describe this process of the mask seeming to have 'a life of its own' which dictates its form.)

*Session 4*

The paint has dried by this session. When Debra looks at the mask she is startled by the sinister effect that the red and black have produced. She states the mask looks like 'a night monster'. She places it on a table and considers the colouring she wants for the lower half. She mixes a dark red from the poster paints and applies this colour to the outlines of the lips. However, she is unhappy with the effect this produces although she is not sure what she wants. When this colour has been removed she tries some silver from a felt-tipped pen, saying that this is more in keeping with the kind of monster she wants to produce. She explains that 'silver, meaningless assurances of safety are spoken from this mouth. This mask will try to seduce and bully the other mask with barren promises.' She feels that the second mask is now complete.

The two masks are placed, side by side, on the table and the therapist invites Debra to name them. She hesitates for a few minutes and then asks if 'the unnamed' can itself be a name. When this is affirmed she volunteers the information that the second mask is named 'The Night Monster with No Name' and the first one is 'The Unnamed Damsel of the Meadows'.

*As she looks at the masks she says she feels the sensation that 'they seem to be part of me yet removed from me'. This enables projected parts of the self to be viewed from varying perspectives and re-examined from a dramatic point of view.*

At the end of this session and all subsequent sessions the masks are placed in boxes and sealed. They will be discussed in greater detail during the next sessions.

*Session 5*

MASK 1: THE UNNAMED DAMSEL OF THE MEADOWS

*A beautiful woman who loves nature and all living things. She dresses in long, flowing robes of green and wears a thin cloak of gossamer red. She does not fear the elements so they never harm her. The sun protects her from its rays, the snowflakes drift safely around her, the rain knows that she appreciates the way it helps the vegetation to grow so it takes care not to drench her. She lives in a reed hut at the edge of a meadow and tends to all wounded animals. She knows the ancient arts of healing and is always ready to help the lame, hurt and orphaned animals.*

*She is young and old at the same time. She has lived here for ever, yet each day marvels at the splendour of the hills, streams and the crops with their abundance of colour and freshness. She is kind but self-sufficient, warm yet independent, giving but not afraid to take the gifts that nature offers her. She changes with the seasons and has no expectations of how the elements should behave at a certain time. She welcomes the sun in winter, the wind and rain in summer and snow in spring. She does not set formulas that cannot be kept to.*

*She knows the patterns of her body will adjust to changes and she will be able to survive by living with the elements rather than expecting them to fit in with the way that people have monitored time.*

*She is as comfortable with night as she is with day. She knows the moon is as valuable as the sun, and the stars have their own kind of brightness. She is as familiar with the animals of the night as she is with the animals of the day. She knows that day will follow night, night will follow day, and so is aware of the patterns of dawn and dusk.*

Debra is slightly bemused by the character sketch she has created. She states that she has never considered the seasons or nature in this way and is not sure that 'any of this' has anything to do with her. She considers this for a while, then states that the description has come from her imagination. The therapist and client discuss this in relation to dreams which can often appear to have 'nothing to do with us' until we examine the symbols they contain in more detail. She agrees that we take time to allow a meaning or insight to form. Meanwhile, she knows that she likes the 'Damsel of the Meadows' and the mask she has made.

Now that the character of healing has been created we can turn to the other mask. As Debra creates the persona for the 'Night Monster with No Name' the therapist ensures that the first mask stays within her sight lines so as to act as a kind of 'safety net' if working on the second mask becomes too uncomfortable or distressing.

MASK 2: THE NIGHT MONSTER WITH NO NAME

*The monster is always covered in a thick gauze which creaks when he moves. He looks like a man but he is really a creature from the swamps that was created thousands of years ago. He is made from slime, clay and rotting trees. The gauze is thick with rotting vegetation and he cannot tell the difference between his body and his clothing. He moves slowly and with intent. He has no feeling for others. He only wants to damage everything around him so he can encourage the rotting process.*

*He moves and speaks like a snake. Beautiful words come from his mouth; he hopes to fool people into his swamp. He will lure any person or animal into the deep mud. He is a bully who wants to crush and defeat anything he sees. He dislikes everything, even the mud in the swamp.*

*During the day he burrows in the mud, eating insects and the roots of any plants that attempt to grow. He slimes and slithers through his evil life, always alone and always trying to destroy anything he can get power over.*

*He dislikes the moon and the stars because they cast light. He wants the silver of his lips to be the only gleam in the night. He uses it to attract his prey. He wants his lips to be the only part of him that is seen. He is a vile and horrible creature, a monster created by the Devil, a thing made from everything horrible.*

At this point Debra is visibly distressed. She is not crying but shows her distress through the tension in her facial and neck muscles. Her breathing has become shallow and rapid. The therapist asks her to look at the first mask and become aware of the flowing movements associated with it. As she becomes more aware of this mask, she is encouraged to transfer the flowing movements on to her own breathing patterns. As she does this her breathing becomes deeper and her tension starts to decrease. Slowly she releases the tension and her distress is alleviated.

Debra is rather surprised that she has become upset by a mask character and again denies that the character 'has anything to do with her'. She says she now feels uncomfortable with the second mask and wishes she hadn't made it. The therapist asks her what she finds particularly uncomfortable about the monster mask. Debra replies in a hesitant way that it is the way he cannot tell which is his own body and which is the gauze that covers him.

After she says this she becomes very pensive and eventually says that she, too, is unsure about her body limits: 'But does this make me bad, too?' When this is reflected back to her she sighs and says, 'I don't do harm to anyone else – that's what makes him bad.' The therapist acknowledges this important statement. The session closes with a repeat of the breathing patterns inspired by the Damsel mask which allows Debra to make positive connections with her body. The masks are placed in their boxes; Debra seals the box containing the second mask with extra layers of masking tape.

*THERAPIST'S THOUGHTS AND REFLECTIONS*

*Debra is taking her phrase 'to create from her own image' in a quite literal manner, especially in relation to the second mask. It will be important to move further into projective work to allow her to work with the masks in a metaphorical way and create a more dramatic distance. As Jones (1995) puts it, 'The process of working through symbol or metaphor will introduce a different perspective on the problem being encountered by the client. The language of metaphor or symbol frees explorations' (Jones 1995, p.235).*

*Time needs to be spent with the first mask before introducing the second mask into a dramatic scenario otherwise Debra could feel chaotic and unable to cope with the power of the monster. Debra may become quite frightened by the power of her imagination/creativity and resort to denial of the masks as products of her own imagination. In essence, the therapist needs to create a safe therapeutic alliance/space to allow Debra to move into dramatic reality without this being a frightening place to be. A place where she can confront her monster.*

### Session 6

At the start of this session Debra is keen to open the box which contains the mask of the Damsel. She says that she had forgotten what she looks like and wants to 'check' her. She takes the Damsel out of the box with great care, smiling as she looks at the mask. She spends a while gazing at it and then puts it on the table. She asks, 'What do we do now, then?' The therapist replies that this is a good time to start to create the mask's movements. She and Debra discuss the starting point for this. As Debra obviously enjoys looking at the mask the therapist suggests that move-ment can be created by keeping the mask in view before actually wearing it. Debra agrees. Thick elastic is threaded through holes pierced in its edges and it is hung on a hook on the wall, level with Debra's face so she can look straight at it.

The therapist tells Debra to try to re-create the breathing patterns that were inspired by the mask during session 5. Moving her feet slowly she starts to create a balanced movement in which her feet touch and leave the ground in turn, in a synchronised way. She is asked to imagine that they feel the soft grass in the meadows. She closes her eyes to do this. Speaking softly, in short sentences, the therapist instructs her to allow the movement to include her whole body – knees, hips, trunk, shoulders, neck, arms, hands – and then to open her eyes and focus again on the mask. Asked by the therapist if she is ready to wear the mask, Debra replies that she feels ready. With great care she places the mask over her face and puts the elastic in place. She looks in the full-length mirror and studies her appearance. When she feels ready she starts to re-create the flowing movements. Wearing the mask enables her to make larger movements and she starts to make progress around the room, the therapist working with her to create the movements of the Damsel of the Meadows. In this way, day and night, the four seasons are gradually embodied in Debra's movements, which become more expansive until they resemble a flowing dance. The therapist offers a range of soft, thin fabrics and Debra chooses a large piece of material for a cloak. She experiments with this until she finds a way of moving which makes the cloak flow around her.

When the therapist notices Debra is starting to become tired, she asks her to make a final movement which will contain the essence of the mask. Debra makes a large smooth turning movement which causes the cloak to billow around her. She removes the mask and places it back on the hook.

Finally, Debra and the therapist sit facing each other. The therapist asks her to say something about how her body felt when she was wearing the mask. Debra is still and takes a while to reply. She says that she felt the 'inside and outside of her body moving together'. The mask gave her a different outside that she was able to respond to. She would like to keep hold of the breathing rhythms and the feeling of connectedness with other parts of her body.

As the session is drawing to a close the mask is placed back in its box, but Debra does not want to close the lid (to allow the mask freedom to breathe, she says). The other box is barely acknowledged. At present, Debra wants to ignore it.

### Session 7

At the start of this session Debra again wants to check the appearance of the mask 'because I forget what it looks like during the week'. However, she has been aware that her breathing patterns have remained deep and even. This has created a feeling of well-being. She has also been more aware of the way her body moves and of its relationship to space.

The Damsel mask is hung on the hook again and Debra creates the flowing movement by turning towards it. When she is ready she places it over her face. The therapist asks her to move around the meadow environment. As Debra does this, the therapist suggests that a wounded animal is approaching and asks her to respond to it. Debra does this slowly and with very gentle movements. She makes the animal feel safe by stroking it and then cradling it in her arms. She goes on to stroking and rocking it. The therapist asks her to find a safe place for the animal. Debra takes it to a corner of the room and mimes building a soft bed from grass. Coming near the place Debra has chosen, the therapist asks how she will heal the animal. In response, Debra makes a large stroking gesture.

At the therapist's request Debra removes the mask and hangs it on the wall hook. The therapist asks about the animal. It is a very young deer, Debra says, which has lost its parents and is being bullied by the older deer. It is very frightened and thinks it has been abandoned because it is ugly. As well as this, it has a large open wound on its side. Debra says she is sure that the Damsel will be able to heal it, however. Debra and the therapist spend some time discussing the form of the healing and Debra agrees to write some suggestions between sessions.

Now Debra thanks the mask for the movement 'it has given her' and 'the ability to think about healing'. When the therapist reminds her of the deer she asks for a box to keep her safe. (Although she has provided a gender for the animal, she continues to refer to it as 'the deer'. The therapist does not comment.) Debra mimes putting the animal in a box, placing the mask's box near it. She moves the new box into a lower shelf in the cupboard.

*THERAPIST'S THOUGHTS AND REFLECTIONS*

*The hurt animal is important and obviously contains some of Debra's own pain. It will be useful to develop this character before moving on to the Night Monster mask which is still, literally, shut up within its box. It may be useful to create an animal mask. To be aware of the possible connections between the animal and the monster, it may be feasible to create these within the story/play, taking care not to force this, however. If the next session is based on a healing ritual, this will lead back to the wounding. Debra is, slowly, becoming more connected with her body through the movement/drama. She has not had the impulse to harm herself during the period of therapy. If she is introduced to the role of playwright, this will increase the dramatic activity.*

*Session 8*

At the start of this session Debra is keen to hang the mask on the wall and look at it for a while. She wants the animal box to remain in the cupboard. She has written some ideas for a healing ritual, but is reluctant to share these with the therapist, saying that she thinks the therapist should be the person to create the ritual because she is 'supposed to be the person who is helping'. The therapist replies that she will co-operate with Debra to create the ritual but it does need to be *her* mask's healing powers that are activated. Debra is quite annoyed by this response and wonders, aloud, whether any of 'this' can be any use or help. Rather than entering into an intellectual dialogue about methods of enabling our own inner strengths and healing powers to be activated by dramatic activity, the therapist asks if she will, after all, share the sentences she has written. Debra agrees, although she is reluctant to produce the paper. 'I have only written about the juice of the grasses, the sap of the trees and the colour of the flowers. There needs to be a big bowl of water for the deer to look at herself in.' The therapist asks about the qualities that the grass, trees and flowers contain. Debra shrugs her shoulders and says she does not know. The therapist suggests that the mask will know and asks Debra to follow her usual course of action for preparing to wear it. It takes some time to focus on the movements but she does eventually recapture them; then she asks the therapist to get the animal's box out of the cupboard before she dons the mask. The therapist puts the box in the same place that Debra had created for the animal's bed during the previous session. Wearing the Damsel mask and cloak Debra moves towards the animal and strokes it. She does not remove it from the box. Keeping the Damsel mask in place she is able to move in a flowing way as she tends to the animal, miming the actions of making it comfortable, by stroking and soothing it. She starts to make a sound – the first – from behind the mask. It is a soft humming, low and repetitive, almost like a lullaby. She mimes collecting the flowers and grasses in a way that suggests she is clear about the purpose of her actions. She goes on humming while she is placing them around the box.

This has taken to within 15 minutes of the end of the session. The therapist speaks to the character she is playing, suggesting that healing needs to be left at this stage for a while. In character, Debra strokes the imaginary creature and puts the box in the cupboard, placing the 'flowers' and 'grass' around it. Slowly she removes first the cloak, then the mask.

Now she is quite still. The therapist helps her to de-role by asking her what she would like to leave behind and what she would like to take with her from the mask character. Debra says she would like to take the feeling of the 'inside and outside of her body working together' and leave behind the idea of 'being someone else'. She places the mask, the 'symbol of being someone else', in the box near the animal.

To close, the therapist asks how the animal feels now. Debra replies, 'OK – safe', and says she would like to 'do a bit more with the animal'. She does not explain further, and the session closes.

*THERAPIST'S THOUGHTS AND REFLECTIONS*

*Has the suggestion of asking her to create the ritual between sessions been helpful or would it have been better to create it within the session, while Debra was wearing the mask? One useful aspect was that Debra was able to express some dissatisfaction with creating the healing herself. At this point, it was probably right to avoid more interaction about this as it would have detracted from the creative aspects of what was happening. In fact, she did not need assistance to start tending to the animal.*

*The meaning of her statement 'do a bit more with the animal' is unclear and will be discussed at the start of the next session. It will probably be helpful for Debra herself to create the role of the animal.*

*She has twice stated that she is feeling the 'union of the inside and outside of her' as a positive aspect of the therapy. It will be useful to check how this is operating within her everyday life.*

*The therapist is aware of her own feelings about wanting to look after the animal as soon as possible and needs to guard against rushing the process. She wonders whether she is, in fact, colluding with the client's avoidance of the Night Monster mask. Further reflection guides her towards the myth of Pandora's Box; but she is aware that in this case she has not had instructions forbidding her to open the box. On balance it seems wiser to work within a healer–wounded–monster sequence. A session with her supervisor helps her to understand that the monster may not be part of the same drama but from another scenario; or indeed, the act of creating the mask and its subsequent containment could be all the work that is required. The supervision session suggests themes of openness and containment to be explored within the drama and the client–therapist relationship.*

*Session 9*

As usual, the therapist checks how Debra is feeling. Debra says that she is conscious of a difference in her relationship with her body and no longer feels 'detached' from it. The therapist guides her towards the statement she made at the end of session 8 about the animal. Debra says she is not sure, but 'feels a pull to know more about the creature'. Because her desire is immediate, she does not seem to need to be channelled through a mask in order to assume the character of the animal. Rather than moving straight into the animal's pain, which does seem to have direct links with Debra's own emotional pain, the therapist suggests that she goes though the ritual of putting the Damsel mask on the wall and connecting with it before she puts it on and sits about tending to the animal as the Damsel. This is what Debra does. She is very tender with the animal, whose box has been placed within the working area.

Now the therapist works with Debra to de-role her from the Damsel character. A bed of cushions is created to represent the animal's own grass bed. Debra is invited to represent the animal by placing herself in the position she imagines it to be. She does this slowly and with precision. She does not try to imitate or impersonate the animal, but to capture its essence. Her breathing becomes shallow and her limbs listless. Her eyes become her major source of expression as she gazes at the Damsel mask, which is on its wall hook. 'What sounds are you making?' asks the therapist. Together, they create a soft, whimpering noise as the creature struggles for breath. These sounds are developed into words and short sentences: 'I am wounded but I feel safe.' 'I enjoy being stroked, it helps me breathe.' 'I know the Damsel will heal me.' 'I will run and play again.'

Now the therapist understands that the animal has faith in the Damsel's power to heal. Therefore she feels it will be safe to explore how the animal became emotionally and physically hurt. She asks the animal to tell the story of her wounding. As the deer, Debra says she cannot remember. 'Please stroke me,' she says. As the therapist has already made physical contact (to which Debra consented), she moves closer to Debra and strokes her shoulder. Debra relaxes visibly and the therapist strokes her back with soft, gentle motions. *She does not take on the persona of the Damsel to do this as it would mean impersonating a character Debra has created without coaching or instruction from her.* Debra, as the deer, allows her breathing to become deeper. The tension in her body disappears. Her eyes close and she makes a soft, contented sound.

As the session is drawing to a close the therapist moves a short distance away from the client in order to enable her to de-role. The mask is placed in its box and returned to the cupboard, followed by the animal box. During the closure Debra expresses love for the wounded animal and feels confident that it can be healed. The therapist does not break the dramatic metaphor by relating this statement back to Debra's own life.

## Session 10

During this session Debra speaks in the character of the wounded deer to tell the story of how she was wounded.

> *The deer remembers her parents being with her and looking after her. One day they went into the forest and did not return. She waited and waited for them but in vain. Eventually she went to ask some other deer what to do, but they laughed at her and told her she was silly. She begged for help but they told her that she was uncoordinated and ungainly, too clumsy to join in their games. She felt lonely and ugly, so she ran away from the place she knew. She was crying as she ran because she thought her body was ugly because she had been told this so many, many times. She started to try to hurt it as the cause of so much taunting. She rubbed her body against sharp twigs. She needed the pain to punish her body. She did not realise that her body and mind were both part of her. She hated her body so much but liked the blood. It was sticky and nice. It looked just like everyone else's blood. It was normal. But then she did not want it to be normal, she wanted it to hurt. So she put nasty things in the cuts. She cried and cried and no one cared. She wanted someone to ask 'What's wrong?' but no one did. But she knew something that no one else did: she knew she was trying to change things by punishing her body.*

Although she is speaking as the deer, Debra uses the third person. The therapist is aware that she is probably speaking about herself through the persona of the deer, but does not attempt to make direct links or challenge the language: to do either would probably stem the flow. At times Debra is quite tearful as she establishes her own insights.

Each time she de-roles with the therapist she is sad to say goodbye to the deer, but feels she is safe because of the Damsel's presence.

## Session 11

Succeeding sessions focus on the healing ritual which Debra creates in the role of the Damsel. Imaginary flowers, grass and sap are placed in an actual bowl brought by Debra for this purpose (a large earthenware bowl). This mixture is placed on the animal's wound which is represented by a brown piece of brushed velvet fabric. The area is surrounded by flowers, each of which has a particular significance. The Damsel asks each flower to grant its healing power to the deer. Daffodils give strength and vitality; roses add their perfume and also give protection from their thorns; violets bring peace and beauty without pride; and sunflowers give confidence in success and the ability to be seen. The Damsel goes to each flower, receiving its gifts for the deer. This ritual is performed four times, at dawn, during the day, at dusk and during the night. Although the ritual remains the same, the Damsel says it needs to be performed at each stage of the 24-hour cycle in order to be effective. After the fourth cycle the bowl of water is produced for the deer to look into.

*At this point the therapist suggests that Debra should resume the character of the deer.*

As the deer, Debra looks into the bowl of water and she says she can see a beautiful face. When questioned, she says that she can feel the wound in her side healing. It is soothed by the balm. She likes the feeling.

The therapist suggests that a round mirror could be substituted for the bowl of water and Debra (out of role) agrees. She resumes the role of the deer and looks into the mirror. She smiles at what she sees.

*Session 12*

The therapist asks whether the deer could look into a full-length mirror. Debra agrees and after assuming the character of the deer, whose wound is now healed, she stands upright and looks into the mirror. After making some fluid movements, she turns to the therapist and says, 'This is my body I'm looking at, you know, and it's OK.'

During the reflective closing of the session she tells the therapist that the Damsel 'is my body too' but the movements were created by the mask.

*Session 13*

During this session Debra thanks the Damsel mask for allowing her to 'discover' her body and make the links between the body, mind, spirit and environment. She also thanks the deer, represented by the velvet fabric, for allowing her to accept the Damsel's healing.

*Session 14*

This session is focused on the Night Monster mask which has, up to now, remained sealed in the cupboard. The therapist is quite surprised by

Debra's response to the idea of looking at it. She takes the box out of the cupboard and unseals it in a very matter of fact way. She places the mask on the table and looks at it without emotion. After a while she says, 'I suppose you don't need to be afraid of monsters you make yourself.' Almost simultaneously she and the therapist recall her earlier request that she should 'make the mask from her own image'. Debra goes on to say that the monster is less frightening out of the box, when he can be seen 'in the open'. The therapist reminds her of her earlier expressions of self-harm as a kind of secret, and how this links to what she is saying about the mask.

They discuss what Debra would like to do with the mask. She says she would like some time to think. Meanwhile, she would like to take the Damsel mask home.

### Session 15

At the next session Debra says that she would like to bury the Night Monster mask so 'he is not destroyed but loses his power which can only exist in the bog. Dry earth will allow him to be turned into a part of the soil.' She wants to bury him in a flower bed 'so he will be a part of a flowering patch and eventually help growth'. This is done during the next session in a local park which has secluded areas. (The season was early winter.)

*The sessions are terminated by a succession of monthly meetings of half-an-hour followed by a three-month break before the final session.*

### Final session

Debra reports that she rarely experiences the impulse to self-harm. When she does she is able to focus on flowing movements either by actually moving or imagining the flow of blood around her body which brings harmony. She says she feels connected to her body and is able to accept herself as she is – 'warts and all', as she puts it. During 'low' periods she is able to ask for physical comfort from her partner or soothe cream into her face in the way she learnt when preparing for the mask work. She has also bought some books on self-massage and is finding the exercises helpful.

She accepts that the impulses to self-harm or to return to self-loathing may return, but she feels that she has learned a way of coping with them.

The following are group exercises involving mask-work, rather than articulated dramatherapy processes.

### 'Monsters'

- Standing in a circle, remind one another of stories, legends and myths involving monsters. Draw a large monster, painting or crayoning it on a big sheet of paper in the centre of the group. Everyone helps to create this image, either directly or by giving directions and advice.

- As individuals, draw an outline impression of one of these monsters' faces on a piece of A4 paper. This should take up most of the space on the paper and be roughly the same size as the artist's own face. Pierce holes in the drawings where the monster's eyes would be, and hold your 'mask' in front of your eyes.

- Walk or run round the room, making appropriate 'monster noises' and trying to scare people. Come together with everyone else, not wearing your mask.

*Discussion: what was it like to pretend to be a monster? Did wearing a mask make a difference?*

### 'Acting the hidden me'

- Group members sit in a circle, facing inwards. Drawing materials have been set out in the middle.

  *Leader:* I'm going to give everybody a sheet of paper. I want us to use the crayons or the paints – or both – to make masks which are big enough to cover our faces. It doesn't matter if you don't think you're any good at drawing or painting, just do your best and that will be good enough.

- Draw a face on your paper which you think resembles your own. Make holes in the paper where your eyes and mouth would be, and hold the mask over your face. Form into pairs and hold conversations with each other. Try to do this as naturally as you can, as if you are not wearing masks (or the group leader may suggest an interesting topic of conversation.) Now join up with another pair, until eventually you're all talking together like this.

- Drop your masks. What was it like, wearing a mask of yourself?

> *Leader:* You've tried out wearing masks which look like the way you think you are. Are there any other ways you think you are? Ways you think you *might* be? We're going to make two more masks. The first of these is a picture of how you'd *like* people to see you.

- Make masks of 'your best side', repeating the stages above. What was wearing this mask like? (This may take longer than the previous similar discussion above.)

- The leader describes the third mask that is to be made – a mask of 'the side of me I am anxious, ashamed or secretly alarmed about and would prefer to keep hidden'.

> *Leader:* You've got a choice here. You can make something up if you want, or you can tell the truth. You don't need to be completely honest, though. It's entirely up to you! Don't forget, it's a mask so no one can really tell what's behind it – except you.

- Repeat the three active stages above, wearing your final masks.

*Discussion: did wearing a mask help you express things about yourself? If it did, then how? Was it easier to be dishonest? Easier to be honest?*

Members can take their masks away with them or simply abandon them. Mask 3 may actually be destroyed *in situ*; however, this must be done only out of sight (e.g. behind a screen) so that other members of the group are unable to see which of the group are holding on to their third mask and which are destroying it.

### 'Family masks' 1

- Using sheets of A4 paper, make outline drawings of the members of a family over three generations – mothers, fathers, children, grandparents, uncles, aunts, cousins – so that everyone is given a different family member. (This can be done by writing the name of the family member on a piece of paper, folding it and inviting people to choose from the pile of papers.) Lay the masks on the ground (or on a table) so that they may be assembled as a 'family group' and people can inspect one another's masks. Take as much time as you want to do this.

- Using the 'folded papers' method described above, take on the character of the person portrayed in a particular mask. Form 'families' of masks and hold conversations 'in character', each family talking among itself. If there is more than one family, families can introduce themselves and their members to one another. What is it like to belong to this particular family? What kind of family would you like to belong to, given the choice? Swap masks and assume different roles. This can happen several times, so that each person has an opportunity to play the part of at least one member of each of the three generations.

- Families decide among themselves which part members will play in a short scenario. This is rehearsed once or twice by the whole family. You may negotiate as to which role you want to play, or think you would play best. Show your scene to the rest of the group, first with the masks and then without them.

*Discussion: the whole process is mulled over by the group, so that people have an opportunity to look at what it felt like to play the role of (a) somebody belonging to another generation; (b) somebody in your own generation other than you; (c) somebody in a family apart from your own; (d) somebody else in your own family. What difference did wearing a mask make? Was it easier or harder to play a scene in front of other people if you were wearing a mask? People are given the change to speak as themselves and 'ordinary reality' is asserted once again before the group disbands.*

More elaborate and substantial masks may be created for these exercises. The advantage of paper masks, however, is that they are very easily produced and this kind of mask work needs to be spontaneous. If a good selection of ready-made masks is available, covering a wide age range, they may be used; but it would be better to spend time deciding on your own mask and then paint it yourself, using one of the blank mask-shapes available nowadays.

## 'Family masks' 2

This is an extension of the previous exercise, in which people use masks to portray their own families. The use of masks allows a good deal of freedom for the expression of feelings about personal relationships which are emotionally highly charged; because it creates a world which is obviously somewhat removed from 'ordinary reality' it relieves some of the pressures belonging to that kind of reality and allows people to think clearly about aspects of their life with other people they usually prefer to avoid.

- The first two stages are the same as in 'Family masks 1'. Prepare sets of masks, representing members of your own families. Have a go at creating 'family portraits' using group members to represent the members of your own family.

- Wearing the mask created by the person whose family you are presenting, speak in role as if you were 'the person of the mask'. This can be done using information supplied for the purpose along with the mask, or simply by looking at the mask and allowing your imagination free rein.

*Discussion: say what it was like to make these masks and see them acted out in this way. Those actually wearing the masks are invited to share their experience with the group.*

Some time is spent de-roling individuals and the group as a whole. What is the difference between mask and reality? People are given the chance to say something about themselves *as* themselves and to describe the way they experience being members of their own families.

# CHAPTER 5

# Into and Out of Chaos

## Dramatherapy and the Symbolisation of Life-Changes

Life experiences that are really new, genuine changes of direction come out of a state of affairs in which the world as it used to be no longer makes any kind of sense for us and needs to be put right in order to 'work' properly again. Putting it right, however, involves remaking it, somehow starting over from the beginning, because simply altering it is obviously not good enough to produce real change in it. This particular state of affairs has gone far beyond the stage at which adjustment is possible. Perhaps if we try really hard we can think of ways in which it could be reordered and the balance of things restored, by paying more attention to this and less to that, by concentrating more on this and teaching ourselves not to care about that at all. We turn out, however, to be more skilful at thinking out solutions than we are at living them.

People who find themselves caught up in this kind of chaos find themselves going over and over the same ground without getting anywhere. No matter which way they turn they end up in the same place. It seems to them that the harder they try the further away they are from reaching any kind of solution to the problem of living. Life goes on at the biological level, but meaning, hope and purpose have long since departed; they feel themselves to be in the same position as Sisyphus, the legendary Greek hero who was destined to spend eternity pushing an immense boulder to the top of a mountain only to have it roll back, time after time, to the bottom. If only something would change – but it never does. The fact is that for human beings life without personal meaning is chaos. If I cannot do things that seem to have purpose, my world falls apart.

Trying to help people in this kind of desperate position is obviously a problem. Somehow something genuinely new has to be introduced into the way they think and feel about life. Rearranging the various elements in their personal chaos will not work. It cannot be made to work, either by them or by anyone else who takes it upon themselves to try and sort things out for them. What they need more than anything else, the only thing that can help them, is *the experience of newness*. The point to be stressed here is that, according to them, there is no way in which this experience can emerge unassisted from the materials provided by their own consciousness; try as they can, they themselves cannot create any pattern within the mind's kaleidoscope. The transformation of chaos must always come from elsewhere.

This, in fact, is what happens. At least it is how they experience this kind of change – as an unexpected deliverance, an experience of being rescued from something entirely overwhelmingly negative. Something intolerable which demands relief. The relief, when it comes, is as powerful as the turmoil, for the two things obviously belong together just as the ending of intense physical pain makes us faint from relief. It is as if this kind of chaos were an actual location, a place we would find no way of getting out of, a cage we were locked into and would never leave. Now, suddenly, we are free. The cage is unlocked, the door is wide open and we are at liberty. The world we find ourselves in now manages to be both new and old. We have never been here before and yet we recognise it joyfully as our own. We discover that to be delivered is to inherit our true identity.

It is never a case of one thing simply growing into something else, something recognisably connected with it so that the new is a logical development of the old. In human experience, to be genuinely, authentically new, something must intervene in order to separate the future from the past, something which is obviously and inescapably different from both so that it cannot under any circumstances be mistaken for or confused with either. For chaos to be chaos it must be total; in other words it must break the rules which govern our experience of time past and time to come, thus contravening every kind of sense at our command so that we are set afloat without map or compass on a sea of confusion and hopelessness.

> Change can only come about when there is a dis-equilibrium in the personality, an imbalance which demands change. The therapist works with the forces engendered by this disequilibrium, his task is to direct them towards a new balance in the personality which will be more

stable because it does further justice to inner needs and the demands of outer reality. (Foulkes and Anthony 1957, p.70)

If we are ever to make landfall we must allow ourselves to be changed in ways that will allow us to start building our lives again – a new kind of life in a world that for us is new and strange, but at least has the priceless benefit of making its own kind of sense. The more complete and destructive the chaos, the more blessed is the experience of reconstruction that characterises its departure. The two things, chaos and deliverance, belong together, each gaining its force from the other. Together they allow us to experience the world as authentically new. 'Life-before-chaos' and 'life-after-chaos' are distinguished from each other by a gap in our experience, a purposeless time in which we are going round and round in circles, getting nowhere at all.

Looking back at the experience, however, we may feel that chaos has a purpose after all, its role being precisely this: to allow a new kind of future to take place by separating it from the past in a way that is clear and dramatic and cannot be misunderstood. To put this in another way, chaos allows the past to die so that the future may be born. This is the meaning of the creation symbolism of many religions which see 'chaos as the womb of life' (Eliade 1958, 1968). In fact, religious symbolism often presents chaos as almost entirely creative. Throughout the world, says Mircea Eliade, a symbolic return to chaos is equivalent to preparing a new creation. Two areas of human life in which this principle is demonstrated very clearly are religious initiation and the rituals surrounding the disposal of the dead – in itself a form of initiation as departed souls are ceremonially incorporated within the world of the dead which is waiting to receive them.

In the middle section of the traditional threefold funeral ritual among the Malekulan people of Polynesia, the dead are taken on a journey which involves traversing a succession of dangerous situations devised to prevent their return to the land of the living, including a maze which is symbolic of the impenetrable confusion that holds sway in the area between the life of this world and the new life that awaits beyond the grave. This pattern of ceremonies is characteristic of many funeral rituals. Everywhere, initiatory ceremonies have institutionalised the experience of chaos by including it within the actual shape of the ritual, where it takes up the central position, a special 'ritual of chaos' surrounded on both sides by ceremonies designed specifically to contain it, and by doing so to separate themselves from each other so that the symbolism of the old state of affairs existing before the initiation ceremony can be set apart totally and dramatically from that of the new, post-initiation world that will emerge as a result of rite. Chaos is the heart of these rituals; the people involved in them are subjected to experiences specifically designed to express and embody a state of affairs without recognisable structure in which life as it was has come to an end without their being, as yet, anything to take its place. Anthropologists such as Arnold Van Gennep (1960) and Victor Turner (1974) have described the unique 'terror of the threshold' that is experienced in between the two outer movements of the threefold structure of rites of passage, in which the characteristic human experience of suddenly finding oneself adrift in a world without recognisable landmarks is created on purpose, specifically to bring about the kind of human experience that can only occur as a reaction to chaos – an experience of deliverance, of being born into a world that *really feels new*. The aim is not to deceive the people taking part, but to involve them in the ritual drama by creating an imagined world in which chaos and deliverance can be lived through and not just thought about (Lewis 1980).

A dramatherapy client said: 'Once you have arrived in the new place, you can look back and remember and use your imagination to relive what happened before – but in order to get to this new place, this really new place, you have to leave the old one behind you. That's the only way you can do it. You can't do it any other way.' Dramatherapy, like ritual, can act as a safe way of containing chaos. We have seen how drama uses imagination to undermine the defences we erect against direct confrontation with the things about ourselves and our lives which trouble and disturb us. The simple business of putting together a drama to express what it is that confuses us and oppresses us, and to use actual people apart from ourselves as a way of embodying these things, is to make them part of a world that is both manageable and an accurate representation of our own personal reality. Dramatherapy presents us with a reality that we can manage, one in which we ourselves set the pace for our own disclosure. Jennings (1990) has drawn attention to the way in which a dramatherapy session reproduces the shape of a rite of passage, and the significance of this with regard to experiences of personal initiation and rebirth has been explored by Grainger (1995) and Duggan and Grainger (1997). As we said in

Chapter 1, the basic dramatherapy process represents the shape of human life-changes: in other words, it has a clear beginning, middle and end, actual change taking place in the middle part of a three-part process. The first part is concerned with a particular state of affairs which has its roots in the past and determines the form taken by our present experience. The third part embodies a new way of being, a new kind of present. In between, things happen that we did not plan and are not prepared for; the use of dramatic structure gives us the chance of experiencing the kind of imagined reality that cuts directly across the one which usually holds us captive, so that things that formerly limited and oppressed us are drained of life. This is a destructive condition to find oneself in, a time and place in which the past has been put to death before the real future has had the opportunity to be born; yet this chaos is the matrix of the whole dramatherapy process, and the secret of its power to produce genuine change in those taking part.

It must be said that not every dramatherapy session produces this effect on the experience of the people involved in it. However, the opportunity to become involved in a shared imaginative experience has a way of loosening the stranglehold of the reality which holds us fixed centre-stage in our own personal life drama, so that even those for whom the world is unbearably chaotic when they arrive for a dramatherapy session find themselves relieved by a form of treatment uniquely willing to take them as they are – one which specialises in the experience of chaos and even values it as the essential condition for the emergence of new life.

For this is precisely what dramatherapy does. Dramatherapists realised that the only way that life can be organised along new lines is by allowing the old ones to remain broken and confused, until new pathways can be established by the person themselves and in her or his own time. In all her work, Sue Jennings urges us to stay with chaos when we find it; and not to try to find explanations for emotional disturbances which, given the opportunity to express themselves in a shared dramatic experience, will sooner or later discover ways of explaining *themselves*, and do so in terms that the person him or herself can understand and do something about. This is what Dorothy Langley (1983) calls 'trusting the method'. It is not as easy as you might think; in fact it takes a good deal of self-discipline on the part of therapists who would much prefer to play safe and plan in advance for anything and everything that could possibly happen. This is an understandable reaction faced with the prospect of having to come to terms with personal chaos – the chaos people bring to a session as well as anything that might occur in it, once people's imaginations are given free rein – but it should be resisted all the same. As we have seen, dramatherapy makes it its business to start from a position of safety; it goes out of its way to establish an atmosphere in which even the most troubled and anxious person present can feel that his or her chaos is understood, accepted and, for the time being, contained. Certainly this means that the first part of any session needs careful planning, special attention being given to the circumstances of each individual and to personal and group histories. In the same way, the final third of each session has a very particular agenda, that of preparing for re-entry into a world that has been temporarily left behind. Even here, however, it is impossible to plan things systematically because of the surprising and unplanned developments that have been taking place in the session itself, within an atmosphere deliberately intended to encourage spontaneity.

It needs to be stressed that it is out of this chaos section of the session that the healing comes, and that this is healing and relief for psychiatric illness as well as release from those states of extreme emotional confusion which accompany any kind of far-reaching and deep-seated personal change and are simply part of the business of being alive, being human. Because of the balance between structure and freedom that characterises all kinds of art-based activity (McNiff 1998; May 1975) and is basic to the arts therapies, dramatherapy has the effect of making disordered thinking and feeling more structured and purposeful while at the same time being able to relieve the obsessional force of depressed ways of looking at the world, when every thought reaches the same inevitable conclusion and life is experienced as static and unchangeable (Grainger 1990; 1995, pp.125–129). For people who are anxious, confused, depressed, emotionally exhausted or numbed by what has happened to them, dramatherapy provides an experience very different from the way of being themselves which they have grown accustomed to and can see no prospect of ever being released from. For a short time during the course of each session they are part of a world that responds to their personhood in a way that is vivid and unforgettable; not simply an idea, but something they actually live through and are able to include in their personal history, not only as *memory* but also as *promise* – the memory of a time and place in which they felt more complete, more human, and the promise that, having happened once, it can happen again.

The chaos envisaged, contained and used in dramatherapy is the same confusion of discordant and conflicting elements that psychologists have recognised as being an essential ingredient of the creative process underlying human perception. To organise the various elements of consciousness is to construct some kind of recognisable human meaning from them. This in itself is a creative action, one undertaken not only by artists but also by every single human being. According to the cognitive psychologist George Kelly (1955), our ordinary problem-solving always involves both a descent into and an emergence from chaos as part of the 'creativity cycle' which 'starts with loosened construction', when things as they are no longer tie up in ways that make sense to us, and 'terminates with tightened and validated constructions', the mind having made new connections which are capable of dealing with the situation confronting it (Kelly 1955, p.528). Any form of psychotherapy that aims to take the facts about the way we make sense of the world really seriously must be willing to see chaos as a potentially healthy experience for human beings. Dramatherapy certainly does this. In Kelly's terms, it can act as the agent of 'validated personal construing' in ways that are vivid, effective and memorable.

To sum up, dramatherapy approaches emotional chaos circumspectly rather than head on. This does not mean that it pussy-foots around, frightened to commit itself to offering the patient any real help, but that the help it provides comes from an unexpected quarter. Emotionally wounded people are very vulnerable to direct approaches, even from those who are eager to help them. It sometimes seems that the more you go forward to meet people who have been psychologically damaged, the more they back away. The reason is obvious, of course. This kind of pain causes defensiveness. We should remember this when we move compulsively forwards to offer help. In dramatherapy, however, the shape of the session, the kinds of activities involved in starting things off at the beginning and drawing them to a satisfactory conclusion at the end, act as a kind of container for the freedom of action and interaction that is allowed to happen in between. If this degree of freedom comes across to people taking part as a frightening absence of structure and stability, the outer framework is there to reassure and support them. Neither the ideas and feelings explored nor the kind of exploration carried out is prescribed;

and the risks that wounded people take in allowing themselves the opportunity for self-discovery and self-expression – for self-actualisation, in fact – are to a large extent compensated for by being able to do so in a safe place among friends. No other approach makes such a systematic effort to provide this kind of security, while making sure that the underlying emotional chaos of wounded and insecure people is not only recognised and respected but also permitted to speak up for itself.

There is a difference, however. The difference between the kind of chaos which disrupts our relationship with everything and everybody, making nonsense of our efforts to live at peace with ourselves, and the chaos presented and lived through during the middle part of a drama-therapy session is simply that which exists between something that cannot be contained and something that can. Dramatherapy chaos, although it certainly feels real at the time (because of its power to remind us of things that for us are only too real), is an experience we not only live through *but also emerge from.* Consequently it can be looked at from another angle. Chaos that is seen from the outside has already lost a good deal of its ability to be really chaotic, at least in the overwhelming and hopeless way that it was before.

The final part of the dramatherapy session is aimed at 'closing chaos off', the intention being to enable those taking part to look back on the experiences of the middle section as an emotional ordeal they have survived, or a problem about life they have managed to solve. This means that although the 'outside world' may not have changed, the way that they feel and think about themselves will almost certainly have shifted. The way that we think and feel about ourselves is the crucial factor in our understanding of the world. It controls the quality of our grasp on reality.

Dramatherapists aim to protect their clients from the threat of personal chaos, ideas and feelings that might overwhelm them so that they can no longer cope with the business of living. On the other hand, it is dramatherapists who are responsible for encouraging their clients to dwell on their own chaos in the first place to the extent of actually performing dramas based on the kinds of thing that cause them the most distress. They do this because they have learned by experience that using imagination in a dramatic way allows us to take our chaos seriously and not turn our backs upon it; because the only way to make sense out of our nonsense is to 'stay with it'.

Within the context of writing about emotional distress we have referred to 'the emotional wound'. This wound may have been with the client since early childhood. The ways in which the wound was inflicted may not be recalled in a clear way, but this does not lessen the aching and pain of the adult consequences of the earlier injury. Vicki Gardiner (1987) and Ann Cattanach (1992) have constructed methods of working with survivors of sexual abuse based on the analogy of the wound, and although the following format for working with survivors does not directly illustrate their work, the inclusion of the wound image was inspired by training undertaken with them.

### Session 1 (connections)

- In a standing circle, allow members to leave as much space as they need between themselves and the person next to them. One group leader holds a ball of thick wool or nytrim. The leader holds the start of the thread and the ball is passed around the circle so a circle of the thread is formed. It is passed around a second time to form a circle of double thickness. The person who started passing the thread secures it by knotting, without cutting, it. The ball of wool/nytrim is then thrown to another person in the group while a verbal connection is made. (This can be any connection from 'I like your shoes' to 'I find your face friendly'.) The person addressed does not respond. Instead, as they catch the ball they pass it around the two thicknesses of thread to secure it, then throw it to another person, making a verbal connection. Continue until a web-like structure has been formed. The group holds the web and pulls it until it is taut. Form different shapes with it. Invite comments about the shape and structure of the web.

- The web is placed on the floor and bags containing small scraps of material are brought into the circle. Invite group members to sort through the fabrics and select some that could represent their feelings of hope (they may be tiny scraps). Return to the web and hold it again within a standing circle. One by one, each person ties a piece of fabric symbolising hope into the fabric of the web.

*Purpose: to provide a structure in which to*

(a) *help the group to establish connections and form the group*

(b) *form a structure resembling a metaphorical safety net*

(c) *act as a symbol of hope for group members to return to when they enter 'the chaos'*

(d) *provide a focus for a ritual opening and closing of the group.*

## Session 2

- The group holds the web. They can add items to the structure, focusing on the symbols of hope. They negotiate an acceptable place in which to locate the web; for example, it may be secured to a wall or draped over furniture. It acts as a reminder of the group connections and the united hopes of the group.

- Group members walk around the room exploring the various textures, areas of light and dark and focusing on the general atmospheres generated by different parts of the room. Do not remain in any area that feels uncomfortable. Gravitate to a place in the room that feels most comfortable. (It may be that there is no area that feels *completely* comfortable.)

- Start to build an environment which will feel safe for group members, using mats, cushions, fabric. (Maybe bring something from home next week.) Each member makes a note of the items they have chosen before dismantling the 'safety area'.

- End by holding the web and making connections with safety.

*Purpose: to establish an actual and metaphorical safe place for group members prior to entering 'chaos'.*

## Session 3

- Start with the web as a focus for the connections that group members may want to make about feelings or thoughts they have experienced between sessions.

- Rebuild places of safety and stay in them. Consider the sources of healing that could be present in this space. Think about the colours and textures used as symbols of hope.

- Using a mask base or a cardboard mask-shaped template, make a Healer's mask. (It will not be worn so it need not be made as a practical mask.) Write about the Healer's powers and character. Place the finished mask within the place of safety (try several positions before deciding where).

- Share information about Healers.

- Close the connections web.

*Purpose: to externalise the inner Healer.*

## Session 4

- Start with the connections web. Exchange feelings, thoughts, experiences in the time between sessions.

- Rebuild safe places and put Healer's mask into position. Spend a few minutes doing this. Reflect on people's need for security – particularly those who have been emotionally wounded as children.

- Find another place in the room that feels comfortable. From a selection of paints, crayons and variety of papers, choose materials to create an image of a wound suffered in childhood.

- Group leader explains the analogy of the wound. Like a wound to the body, emotional wounds may scar the surface and yet remain unhealed at a deeper level. As participants draw or paint, they consider their own emotional wounds which have been left unhealed. Is the edge smooth or jagged? Is the wound deep or shallow? What kind of residue has been left? (The image does not need to be medically correct.)

- Share the images with other group members.

- Close by referring back to the connections web.

*Purpose: to introduce memories and feelings of chaos within a structure of safety.*

**Session 5**

- Open with connections web.

- Rebuild areas of safety and position Healer's mask.

- Spend some time in the safe place. Recall and revive images of the wounds. Are there similarities and differences in the wounds? Using plaster of Paris bandage and paints, create a group model of a shared wound. View this from different perspectives before returning to the safe places to see how it looks from there. Consider the journey from the wound to the Healer. Clear away the images and group wound to keep until they are needed again.

- Use the connections web to sum up and say goodbye.

*Purpose: to externalise and project individual and group feelings.*

**Session 6**

- Remind people that this is the halfway stage of the group.

- Open with the connections web. Restore safe places and Healer's mask. Spend some time in the safe place as a group. Reflect on individual images and the group wound.

- Each person has a ball of thick wool or nytrim. Use this to 'lay out' a journey from individual wounds and the group wound to the healing mask.

- Mark some of the areas on the journey as particular parts of the terrain. For example, the bog of despair, the valley of shame, the forest of fear. Draw a map so the journey can be re-created. View your journey from the place of safety. Reflect on the help the Healer can offer.

- Dismantle journey, images and group wound. Close the connections web.

*Purpose: to create a metaphorical journey from emotional pain to healing.*

**Session 7**

- Start with connections web and set up places of safety and masks. Re-create your journey.

- Stand by group wounds, looking towards safe place and Healer. Focusing on Healer, move towards one of the parts of the journey you have marked. Each person shares with the group the terrain they are in. How does it feel to be in this place? Each person, in turn, speaks about the place they are in. *(Example: 'I am in the vale of shame. This is a lonely place where I shed tears, alone and isolated. It is surrounded by hills, so no light reaches the place. It is desolate and dark. My body curls up and no one can reach me. I feel so alone and ashamed.')* Allow each person enough time to speak at their own pace and express their feelings.

- Using a range of art materials, each person creates an image of themselves within this place. (In the above example, the art work would show a curled-up figure in the dark valley.)

- When the art work is completed, participants form pairs. They discuss their images and swap pictures. One of the partners takes on the role of Healer. They take time to create what they feel to be an appropriate posture within the safe place. (The masks can be held.) When the Healer is ready, their partner approaches them with the picture they have made and explains that a traveller is stuck in the place shown in the picture. The Healer either performs a healing ritual for the traveller or talks about the healing process. When the Healer has finished, the pair change places so that the person who brought the picture now takes up the position of the Healer, performing the ritual or saying the appropriate words. The person who is holding their picture accepts the healing.

- What has this felt like? Holding the connections net, say how it has been for you.

- Pack away materials and images, dismantle places of safety.

*Purpose: to enable participants to discover and activate their own sources of healing.*

**Session 8**

- Start with connections web and reflect on the part of the journey you travelled in the last session. Take time to re-create places of safety and redraw your journey map.
- Repeat format of session 7, each person focusing on a different terrain. This may contain elements of the terrain from session 7.
- Close as session 7.

*Purpose: to consolidate the work done in the last session and the embodiment of the Healer.*

**Session 9**

- Start with connections web. Remind group of the number of times they will be meeting like this. Reflect on journey.
- Re-create journeys and places of safety. Focus on any feelings of 'stuckness' or places that seem to be too difficult to be overcome. Work together to find a common image of such a place; for example, the common image might be of a large bog, in which case some people may want to add elements of raging fire or unscalable mountains to the general picture. Devise ways in which these elements could be added. Discuss whether the image is of the present state of affairs or of the future?
- In places of safety write or draw a message from the healing mask. Read out these messages. Change masks so that another person can read the mask's message to its creator. Write the image or message from the mask onto a small card and decorate it with healing images (e.g. flowers, stars, rainbows). Group members take these away with them.
- Close with connections web.

*Purpose: to focus on the future and the continuation of self-healing.*

**Session 10**

- Start with connections web. Re-create journey and places of safety.

- Focus on a place in the journey that has been conquered or travelled through in safety. Encourage group members to create places that have not been indicated on the journey but that they have travelled through. For example, places of hopelessness, isolation etc.

- Draw or write about this journey and the qualities that helped the traveller to overcome the obstacles on it.

- Each member shares their experiences with others, so that the strength, courage and ingenuity shown can be received and validated by other people. The group takes time to talk about how these strengths can help them in the future.

- Close with connections web.

*Purpose: to move towards closure by reminding each individual in the group of his or her inner strength.*


## Session 11

- Start with connections web. Remind group that this is the penultimate week. Re-create places of safety and the journey.

- Group participants make themselves comfortable in the places they have made safe for themselves. (They may need to add cushions.) After a period of relaxation, the facilitator starts the following visualisation based on the healing mask:

    *Allow the soft colours from the mask to flow around you like a gentle, comforting light. Allow it to flow around your body, bringing comfort and a feeling of safety. Breathe in the light and allow it to flow around the inside of your body. Imagine the light surrounding the image of your wound. Allow the light to flow around the wound and focus on the journey you have taken. Imagine the light healing the wound and focus on the cleansing that the light brings.*

- Following the visualisation, each person creates an image of a healed wound. (This may be further than the stage they have reached in the group.)

- Share these images. Each person states their relationship to the healed wound and their original image of their own wound.

- The group may make any changes they want to the group wound. This may involve adding more plaster of Paris to change it, melting it by adding water to the original so it dissolves. (Violent methods of de-constructing it should be avoided at this stage of the group.)
- Close with discussion about the journey and the healing. What kinds of strengths will people use in the future?
- Repeat connections web exercise as a way of saying goodbye (e.g. 'I have appreciated this connection with you...'). Discuss the possibility of follow-up sessions.

*Purpose: to reinforce images of healing, and of the healing journey undertaken by the group.*

## Session 12

- Take connections web apart. Suggest people might like to keep the fabrics or part of the web. The web still exists even though it is in parts.
- Build places of safety. Draw an image of the place of safety to keep. Then dismantle the places of safety.
- Place pictures of the journey on the floor and write about it. Dismantle the journey; what would participants like to do with the pictures?
- Connection goodbyes, as in previous session.
- Decide on dates of follow-up sessions. These are needed to reflect on the journey while slowly disengaging from the group.

*Purpose: to mark the end of these sessions.*

This form of group is particularly useful for people who have already received some individual therapy/counselling. As it involves masks and the concepts of places of safety as well as the chaos of the journey, it should not be used with people who have not engaged in any prior exploration of their abuse.

## Evaluation

*Therapists keep a journey map for each client as an indication of their responses and feelings during the journey. Clients evaluate in the same way.*

# CHAPTER 6

# What Does It All Mean?
## Dramatherapy and the Interpretation of Life

Ideas and feelings, when they are shared, may grow in intensity until they represent much more than any one single individual would be willing to take responsibility for. In this way 'the group' and what it stands for begins to dominate the people that belong to it. Unfortunately, folk may end up less free than they were before they joined, and less able to exercise their own independent judgement so that they feel in control of their own personal lives. Looking at it this way we immediately think of things like religion and some kinds of party politics or social action which suddenly become the most vitally important things in life for large numbers of people. Sociologists describe a kind of knock-on effect, according to which shared ideas produce group cohesion and cohesion strengthens and validates the ideas that produce it, thus establishing them as 'social reality' (see Berger 1967).

To say the least, this is unlikely to happen in small therapy groups. Here, people gain strengths from being with people they have come to know and trust, and the strength of the group itself feeds back to give courage to the individuals who belong to it – the courage to be *themselves*, not simply group members. Groups function as laboratories for personal development. Another way of saying this would be to talk about the development of meaning. In this context we are not thinking simply about intellectual understanding, however, although the kind of meaning associated with the experience of being a member of a therapy group does help people find relief from the pressure to find answers to problems that present themselves in intellectual form as actual questions: what is it all about? Or – even more urgently – why me? But this kind of question is certainly not just an intellectual query. It goes much deeper than that. It has to do with the way things feel, what it is like to be alive. So it can come from a lack of confidence in actually being alive at all, which can feel quite serious. Certainly it denotes the presence of anxiety, but it should never be dismissed as a mere indicator of a psychiatric condition. It does more than reveal anxiety, because it describes what kind of anxiety it is – what a person is anxious *about*.

People may be anxious about being themselves. About being people. They do not feel the way they think a person ought to feel. Feeling and thinking are mixed up together in this, as in everything else about being human. How I feel about myself is mixed up with how I feel about other people, and how I feel they feel about me. Somehow, I sense that being human is basically about this – about my relationship with other people. It is about reaching out and being reached out to. It is about between-ness (Buber 1957; May 1975; Winnicott 1971).

This is what Jennings means when she talks about the strange ability of groups to promote individuality and co-operation *at all times*: in a group, she says, I am most myself and most together with others. Working and playing – sometimes just being – as a member of the group gives me a special kind of freedom which I can use in two ways: either to be alone in the group or, in fact, to be the group, able to say *we* think, *we* feel, it is *our* opinion, or no thanks, not me if you don't mind, leave me out of this.

Another way of saying this is that the group has the effect of making me feel creative. This is a word that tends to put people off a bit because it is so often used to refer to what is known as 'talent', particularly to those who have an awful lot of it. Beethoven, Shakespeare, they were creative, not me. This is not what dramatherapy means by creativity, however. Being creative means setting out to discover meaning in things. It is something that people do most of the time, whenever they feel confident enough to do it, in fact. Whenever we think, speak or work with a definite personal intention, *really putting ourselves into it*, we are being creative. The psychologist Seymour Sarason (1990) has pointed out that this kind of personal presence in what we do or say is the thing that makes a job of work into a work of art: work and artistic activity are on the same continuum. Nothing has been more effective in obscuring the presence of artistic processes than the tendency to regard them as special features of special people (Sarason 1990, p.2). Creativity is something that belongs to being human. It is natural and basic. People express what they feel about life in the way they express themselves (and vice versa, of course).

Doing things 'for fun' is particularly creative because it allows this kind of freedom of expression. People who certainly do not think of themselves as artists of any kind enjoy a holiday from their own and other people's expectations about what they should do and be by making pictures, dancing, acting things out. This is what I feel about life, says the picture, dance or drama: thank you for letting me show you! (Not bad, am I?) Looked at like this, doing things for fun can be a great encouragement for being creative in other directions, too. It can help us make sense of the whole business of living. Our ham-handed efforts at producing works of art (we would not dream of calling them that) are expressions of a basic urge to give shape and meaning to life.

Some psychologists and psychotherapists understand this very well. Describing one of his clients, the child of a broken home, May (1975) says, 'You can live without a father who accepts you, but you cannot live without a world that makes some sense to you.' He points to what he calls 'a passion for form' in everybody's life that expresses itself at the most personal level in all our relationships (May 1975, p.127). Form, shape, meaning all add up to the same thing, a world we can find our way in, whose landmarks are recognisable to us, whose roads and pathways are kind to our feet, whose barriers – natural or human-made – we know how to set about trying to surmount. In such an environment we are emotion-ally at ease; out of it we will always be to some extent uneasy, if not in real personal distress.

Health and meaning are inextricably bound up together. Emotional health might be described as the process whereby we give meaning and significance to our life stories and the things that happen to us during them. Gestalt psychologists identify the process of healing emotionally disturbed people with the action of re-establishing contact with the environment; to make contact is to make sense. When we are unable to organise our experience of things and people in order to come to grips with whatever is going on around us, we feel psychologically threatened and emotionally disturbed, says Jennifer Mackewn (1997, p.64), because 'awareness and contact are the natural means by which people develop and grow'. 'A passion for form.' Making, doing, being, *actually knowing you exist*; all involve a feeling of completed action of some kind or other. Anxiety and a sense of formlessness and meaninglessness go together. We are aware of a situation in which things fail to 'fit together' for use, so that nothing seems whole or achieves completeness. We cannot really get to grips with life because it is too shapeless. Our dance, drama or picture, because we have made them, stand out for us as evidence of reality, their own and ours. It is possible for things that we have 'made up' to be real; we know they are real because they are *there*, we have made them. We have actually *finished* them! Fritz Perls (1948), the founder of Gestalt psycho-therapy, drew attention to the way in which art, drama in particular, deals with the 'unfinished business' of living. Emotional problems 'cry for solutions, but if they are barred from awareness, neurotic character formation will be the result' (Perls 1948, p.573). As we pointed out at the beginning of this book, dramatherapy does not simply give people scope for creativity; because it is in itself the shape of a work of performance art, simply taking part in it is a way of being involved in the kind of completeness that art symbolises. It can be effectively used for all situations involving the anxiety of unfinished business.

Psychotherapists who work in the humanist tradition, such as Victor Frankl (1964), have always argued that there is an impulse towards personal fulfilment which is innate in human beings, and that this necessarily involves the search for meaning. We are drawn towards meaning 'like iron filings towards a magnet'. Here again, meaning is not simply a kind of intellectual understanding, something confined to our cognitive awareness. It is more instinctive than that, more global: for example, we can all produce sound logical arguments to explain the love that children have for their parents, but when it comes down to it, most people tend to say something like 'because we know it's right' or 'because it *feels* right'. For them, the meaning of family love is simple because this is the best way to be a family.

Obviously there is a difference between family ties and those which exist in a therapeutic group, not only in intensity but also in quality. All the same there are certain similar ties. Groups are known to revive some of the feelings of attachment associated with and first learned in families, and some of the resentments too. One thing we certainly draw upon from our family background is a sense of belonging together; even if we belong to a 'dysfunctional' family, we still tend to feel loyalty to it, as we discover when somebody criticises it and we feel that they are really criticising us too. This, in turn, relates to the difficulties encountered by the group and its individual members and the way these have been overcome. Suffering of one kind or another bonds people together – not only in the present but for the past and future too, as the memory of it forms part of a shared history, a kind of 'family tradition' of the group. Therapeutic groups are primarily concerned with suffering. You could say they were part of an attempt to find meaning in suffering.

We are using meaning here to stand for whatever it may be that possesses the highest value for a person either as an individual or as a member of the group. For example:

- love and friendship

- religious aspiration; relationship with God

- social justice and human rights

- political freedom and freedom of speech

- personal integrity

- family ties

- group and sectional loyalties

- patriotism

- peace on earth

- compassion for suffering, and so on.

These values and others like them attract the kind of devotion that Paul Tillich (1958) has called 'ultimate concern'. They are the source of life's meanings, things that are in themselves worth suffering for. Put simply, they are the most important things in someone's life, with the power to make other things important through association with them. Their meaning rubs off on our lesser concerns.

Making a list of things people pay allegiance to does not actually help us all that much. Meaning is not something that can be categorised in such an obvious way. It is subtler and more pervasive than that. If it can be located anywhere at all, it is 'between' and 'within': between people and within people's lives. In other words, it is interpersonal and existential. We think of it in terms of pictures and mental images which symbolise its meanings for us. Existential images seem to take place *within* us. They are to do with the way we imagine ourselves 'in ourselves'. For example, if we think of ourselves engaged in striving towards a goal, getting deeper into the unknown, suffering defeat or achieving victory, we make contact with the emotional reality of these ideas by seeing them as pictures, or even more vividly as situations we are in, *places where we are* – roads, woods, pits, morasses, spaces, oceans. *Our* pits, *our* oceans and woods. Interpersonal symbols include others; they are images of the way we relate to people and animals, particularly ones we feel strongly about. (When we avoid putting our feelings into words for ourselves, these inner pictures show up just as clearly, perhaps more clearly than ever.) We have images of reaching out and people reaching out to us; journeying to meet someone or having to say goodbye to them, being welcomed, being shunned; fathers who punish us, mothers who 'make us better' (or the other way round, of course); powerful people who bully us and others who let us be ourselves in their company. These, again, are *our places*. We can share them by letting others in on them, but they originate in our experiences of other people and bear the stamp of those uniquely personal experiences.

The connection between the things we stand for and believe in, and their existential and interpersonal images is fundamental: these things cannot be separated. It is these images that give life and power to our enthusiasms, preventing ideas like 'social justice' and 'personal integrity' from becoming mere slogans and catchphrases. At this level of personal involvement my opinion as to what – so far as I am concerned – constitutes the most important thing in the world, the only thing able to make sense of life, is the sign not simply of party loyalty but of spiritual awareness.

Spirituality and religion are not the same, although it would be difficult to be a spiritually aware person without acknowledging that there are some values in life which transcend all other considerations. Most people, however, when they speak about religion, would agree with Brian Thorne (1997) that the word means 'a set of beliefs or understandings which are held in common and attempt to explain, at least partially, the totality of human experience.' Spirituality, on the other hand, does not set out to *explain* anything at all. It simply does not refer to that sort of meaning. Spirituality is understanding by participating. To quote Thorne again: 'It is the experience by which the human spirit shares in the creative source of energy which reflects the moving force within the cosmos' (p.206).

The most characteristic way that human spirituality expresses itself is in the form of myth. Myths are stories of great personal and social resonance, in which human meaning – the meaning of being human – is enshrined. Myth uses human story-making to crystallise our perception of an understanding that is incalculably wider and deeper than our individual awareness and yet relates to that awareness in the truest and most authentic way imaginable. Myth unites my own meaning to the meaning of life. According to Henry Murray (1960), myths involve 'the passionate participation of all functions of the personality (*individual* myth) or of all members of a society (*collective* myth)' (1960, p.335). David Fernstein and Stanley Krippner describe it as 'the primary though often unperceived psychological mechanism by which human beings navigate their way through life' (1989, p.4). In myth, the individual and the social meet in order to face whatever may be beyond.

Dramatherapy provides the framework for a potentially endless succession of mythic images which permit us to explore the spiritual dimension of life. Because it is founded not in words and explanations but in actions and events embodying the presentation of interpersonal truth, it continually suggests ways in which we can give new life to ideas that are vitally important to us and which express our personal meaning, by refreshing ourselves at the source of our commitment to them.

Sometimes dramatherapy starts from myths and legends, as archetypal expressions of human meaning. Often, however, it simply concentrates on things that happen in our ordinary lives and allows the deeper, symbolic, mythic significance to arise out of this quite ordinary, everyday material and present us with a mythic theme to explore and inhabit. In this way drama brings us into contact with interpersonal, existential truth at its most profound, our individual strengths and weakness bound up together in the living imagery of personal relationship which is the source of all human meaning.

Put like this it sounds rather alarming. And yet it does not alarm the people taking part. Freely embraced as a way of expressing what we ourselves have known and felt, these 'frightening' stories provide vulnerable people with a way of reaching out to one another for the personal contact which alone can refresh and restore their lives. The reason is that these symbolic stories are all metaphors of a search for meaning in life that is both individual and corporate, intensely personal and private, and yet characteristic of the entire human race. And dramatherapy clients have shown themselves to be the most appreciative of this fact.

Dramatherapy takes metaphors and word pictures very seriously, particularly when they come from patients. To psychiatrists and people who have become accustomed to the way they think and talk, this must seem a strange thing to do. Not that patients' imagery is without significance to psychiatrists for diagnostic purposes; however, orthodox psychiatry is mainly concerned with images as indications of illness. In other words, a psychiatrist is trained to pay attention not to what a patient's word pictures mean to the patient, or what they are intended to convey to everyone else, but to the simple fact that she or he is making them. Word pictures are not always easy for anyone else to understand, of course. For one thing, they may not be saying what other people expect to hear or, more to the point, perhaps what they are willing to listen to. For another, *they are not easy for the person they belong to to express in any other way.* That is why they are word pictures rather than straightforward descriptions.

People want to say something but cannot find the words to say it, or perhaps they just do not want to say it 'in so many words'. In fact this is very likely to be the case, because what they feel they need to talk about is very painful to them, a source of real personal anguish, so that it is hard, if not actually impossible, to find any words at all. At the same time there is a powerful urge to share, to spread the load, to get the message across and draw attention to the problem; even more, to find someone who can take the pain away. Sometimes even admitting this is painful because we feel that we should not ask for help. There is a definite sense that what we are complaining about is our own fault. Physical illness may be different; we do not necessarily feel we have to blame ourselves for the things that go wrong with our bodies, although we can and often do take the blame for having somehow exposed ourselves to this or that source of danger, so that we now have to take the consequences of our own foolishness. With emotional illness of almost any kind, however, self-blame seems to be obligatory. We feel that our emotions are solely our own responsibility. Our pain may be real – indeed we know it *is* real; nevertheless we should be able to cope with it. We are, in fact, guilty for not being able to deal with what everybody knows is our own business.

Thus an emotionally ill person has a sense of being both victim and perpetrator, a fact that tends to increase the private nature of psychological pain. If what I am going through is my fault, and I am the only one who can do anything about it *and I cannot*, then I will not be very eager to lay myself open to having the fact brought home to me by you. People who feel like this often use indirect ways of getting their meaning across. The truth about themselves that they reveal in what they say and do can be both vivid and unexpected. It is its unexpectedness that sometimes baffles therapists – as, in a way, it is intended to do. The aim is to achieve instant understanding or none at all. The image is vivid and precise, but the therapist must be on the ball to receive it. The alternative is for their patients to have to explain precisely what it is that is troubling them, and to run the risk (which feels more like a certainty) of failing to do so yet again.

Hence the use of metaphor, which is both a way into understanding and communication and a barrier against the wrong kinds of understanding – the kind that other people use to categorise and control me – and the even more punishing awareness with which I manage so successfully to enslave myself. 'Metaphor helps a patient to come as close to his true feelings as he dares' (Cox and Theilgaard 1987, p.9). The more poetic the metaphor is, the better it carries out its dual task of protection and exposure: poetic metaphor 'carries a particular affective loading' which 'resonates with that within the patient which is called into existence' (Cox and Theilgaard 1987, pp.5, 23). This is because our poetic imagination is able to connect our personal pain to our sense of the hidden meaning of life in a way that nothing, except poetry, can. Poetry is both intensely personal and wholly universal. To discover that someone else's core experience of being human is also our own – or at least that it touches us exactly where we hurt, the hidden point at which we most need understanding and acceptance – provides the sense of healing intimacy that we crave. With intimacy comes connectedness. To discover that what hurts us so much, the very thing that cuts us off from other people and makes us feel different, rejected, inferior, hopeless, is in fact the pledge of our belonging, not to a medically marginalised subgroup of society but to the universal human race, dignifies our suffering in a way that nothing else can.

This is something that we have to discover for ourselves. Therapy may be able to set the scene for this kind of revelation, but it can never actually cause it to happen. One of the main strengths of dramatherapy is its ability to handle metaphor and imagery in a restrained way, without imposing it as a kind of ready-made 'answer to life's problems'. The insight that comes from this kind of 'poetic recognition experience' comes spontaneously, or even accidentally. This is mainly because of the metaphors themselves which are usually taken from the material presented to the group by its members rather than predetermined by the therapist before the session begins. Apart from workshops devoted to exploring specific life-themes or concentrating on the use of dramatherapy in various social, medical or institutional contexts which are usually planned in advance, drama-therapists prefer to work in as open a way as possible, establishing the overall shape of the session with as much clarity as they can but letting the things that happen within it emerge from the material that members of a group of actual clients actually bring along themselves.

The following example is a 13-week, 1½-hour group structure based on the Grail Legend.

## Session 1

*Group culture and group rules*

- Names: in a seated circle each person says his or her name. Still in the circle, names are repeated but this time each person gives a short history or description or connections with their name. (They may know the meaning of their name, make connections with family members or fictional characters who share their name.) When everyone has spoken, other group members are invited to make their connections with each other's names.

- In pairs, consider the importance of names. For example, what impressions do people form when they are aware of someone's name before they meet?

- Discuss in large group.

- Goodbyes.

## Session 2

*Warm-up*

- Greetings. Remind people of names by another name round.

- Make a circle of names in alphabetical order.

- Move the chairs to the sides of the room. The whole group makes the shape of the first letter of each person's name. For example, for a person named Susan the group members arrange themselves to form the shape of the letter 'S'. This is repeated for each group member.

- These shapes are then repeated, starting with the first shape. Everyone is invited to look at the shape from the viewpoint of where they are standing or imagine the whole shape. What else could the shape represent? ('S' could be a snake, a winding path, a stream, a silk scarf etc.) Repeat each shape, taking time to consider what it could represent.

*Main activity*

- Walk around the room. Start to create different shapes in response to items suggested by the group leader:

    (a)  A person warming herself by a fire. Feel the heat on the hands, face, body.

    (b)  Someone in a very comfortable position in bed. One of those mornings we just don't want to get up because the bed is so comfortable. Feel the warmth and comfort.

    (c)  Someone sunbathing on a perfect beach. The heat of the sun is just right and we can really relax!

    (d)  A person sitting in a very comfortable armchair. It's been a hard day and it's wonderful to sink into the comfort of the chair.

- Discussion: reflections on comfort – what it means to different people. Encourage other suggestions for comfortable places.

- Walk around the room, noticing other people in the group. Slowly start to make gestures of comfort towards other people. Touch only if this is agreed with the other person.

- In pairs: one person adopts a position of someone in need of comfort, and the other supplies the comfort in a non-verbal way. Repeat with reversed roles. Find other ways to portray the two positions.

- Form threes and repeat the above exercise with one person to be comforted by the other two. Choose one of the images you have created in this group and re-create it in slow motion, paying attention to every move and gesture. Repeat this, adding a few words. Don't spend time creating a scenario, instead focus on creating a moving image. Add a few words that complement the gestures.

- Each group shows their moving image to the others. After each image the entire group offers their perceptions of what the scenario could be.

*Discussion: on receiving and giving comfort.*

*Closure*

- Reflections on the drama. How did playing the different roles feel?
- Goodbyes.

*Purpose: to encourage different perspectives on situations. To encourage different body movements. To enter into dramatic scenarios.*

## Session 3

*Warm-up*

- Greetings.
- Walk around the room shaking hands with other people as they walk past.
- Form two lines, one at each end of the room. Walk slowly towards the person facing and extend your arms in a gesture of greeting. People meet each other in the centre of the room. Repeat a further three times.

*Main activity*

- One of the ways we tend to comfort people is to offer them a drink. In Britain this is often in the form of a cup of tea. Is this familiar to people? Are there other cultures represented in the group? What is their equivalent?

- In groups of three or four, devise a short scene showing the cup of tea (or other representation) being given. Focus on: where, who, when, why, what is happening while preparing the scene? Use the gestures created in the images in session 2.

- Share these scenes with other groups.

- De-role.

*Closure*

- Reflect on the dramas created.

*Purpose: to extend the dramatic capabilities of group members. To put the grail concept into an everyday context in order to ground the reality of the legend.*

## Session 4

*Warm-up*

- Greetings.

- Walk round the room in your usual way and then form a standing circle.

- Imagine that you are generating comfort in the centre of the circle. Focus on generating it right into the centre. If there was a symbol of the comfort created in the centre, what would it be? Work towards a consensus of opinion on what this symbol would be. (It is possible to have more than one symbol if agreement cannot be reached.)

- Focus more comfort into the symbol(s) to regenerate it (them).

- Relax. Now create gestures of taking comfort from the symbol.

*Main activity*

- In small groups of three or four, discuss symbols of comfort. Create a dramatic image of these symbols by group members 'becoming' the symbols; or creating group sculptures conveying the symbols and people's reactions to them; or focus on the giving and taking of comfort from the symbol.

- Focus on the idea of a very special cup which is revered. Create a ritual which has the cup as its focal object. (The word 'cup' can be interpreted in as wide a manner as you wish.) Music can be added if the group wants to.

- Share the created rituals with other groups or incorporate other people into the ritual.

*Closure*

- Reflect on 'giving' and 'taking' and the dramas/rituals created.
- Goodbyes.

*Purpose: to move into ritual prior to the Grail Legend. To explore the concepts of 'giving' and 'taking'. To focus on concepts of symbol and ritual and the meanings of these to group members.*

## Session 5

*Warm-up*

- Greetings.
- Walk around the room easing tension in your body. Start to weave in and out of other people. As other people are passed, say the name of a person from a legend, myth or fairy tale. (The names can be varied, or some people may choose to repeat the same name several times.)

*Main activity*

- In a seated circle, reflect for a few minutes on the names spoken and heard.
- Verbally brainstorm the kinds of quests that were undertaken in the legends/stories.
- Group leader tells the Grail Legend. (How this is told will depend on the group culture and levels of understanding.) The general outline is as follows:

    *The Grail is a mysterious, life-preserving and healing vessel guarded by a king and his court in a castle that is difficult to locate. From this*

*hidden place the Grail calls seekers to undertake the difficult journey
or quest.*

*The king is ailing, lame or ill and his kingdom is a wasteland. The
king's health can only be restored if a hero of considerable substance
locates the castle and then asks a specific question when he witnesses the
Grail and the king. The question is usually, 'What ails thee?' If this
hero fails to ask the question the hero will be expelled from the castle
which will vanish, leaving the hero to resume the quest. If the hero
should succeed, after many adventures, in finding the castle again, and
if he then asks the question, the king will become fertile and the hero
will become the new guardian of the Grail.*

*The Grail itself has been described in various ways, as the legend
has been rewritten and retold over the centuries. Some writers have
described it as a chalice or cup, some as a stone.*

- Group members sit quietly for a minute and reflect on what their image of the Grail is. Each person is given a sheet of paper, with paints and crayons available, and each creates a painting or drawing of the Grail. When these have been completed they are shared with other members of the group and the qualities that each Grail possesses are explained.

- In pairs, discuss the place where both Grails are kept and the kind of ritual/ceremony that takes place when it is taken into the court. These ceremonies/rituals are fed back into the main group.

- Leaders ask people to bring a glass, cup or object that is close to their representation of the Grail.

*Closure*

- Reflect on the Grails and ceremonies that the group has created.

- Goodbyes.

*Purpose: to enable group members to engage with the legend. To start with the
spiritual, positive aspects of the Grail before embarking on the quest. To allow each
person to create their own symbols of healing and regeneration.*

## Session 6

*Warm-up*

- Greetings.
- Walk around the room releasing tension.
- Recall the ritual/ceremony created in session 5. Begin to move in the way that one of the characters engaged in the ritual would move. Extend this movement. Imagine the kind of clothing that would be worn. How will this influence the movement?
- What is the person's relationship with the Grail? Show this relationship within the movement.
- Relax, shake your body and return to your usual way of walking.

*Main activity*

- Group members place any items they have brought on to a table. Those who have not been able to bring an object may choose from a selection assembled by the leaders.
- Grails are created by using plaster of Paris bandage or similar mixtures pasted around or added to objects. A selection of 'gems', glass, paints and spray paints are also available. Allow at least half-an-hour for making the Grails and then put them in a safe place to dry.
- Reflect on the process of making the Grail. What kind of shape is it taking? What did it mean to make the Grail?

*Closure*

- In a circle: what will each person be taking with them from the experience of making the Grail?
- Goodbyes.

*Purpose: to actualise the Grail. To create a meaningful dramatic property as the focus of drama. To extend creative skills. To focus on the Grail, the purpose of the quest.*

## Session 7

*Warm-up*

- Greetings.
- Walk around the room, releasing tension. Allow your body to feel relaxed and balanced. Imagine that the energy from the Grail is flowing around your body and creating a warm, glowing feeling.

*Main activity*

- Each person locates their Grail and holds it. Sense the kind of energy that the Grail emits.
- Divide into two groups. Each group devises a ritual for each Grail. Each ritual is then shown to the other groups. They may or may not be given a definite place in your ritual (for example, as part of a procession or circle).
- Put the Grails in a safe place around the edges of the room.
- In pairs, create a picture of the wastelands.
- Reflect on the pictures and the differences between the energy of the Grail and the wastelands.
- Put the Grails and the pictures in a safe place.

*Closure*

- Reflect on the purpose of rituals and their healing purposes.
- Goodbyes.

*Purpose: to experience the difference between concepts of the barren wasteland and the healing properties of the Grail and its rituals.*

## Session 8

*Warm-up*

- Greetings.
- Say hello to others as you walk around the room. Extend warm, friendly greetings to others. Slowly make the movements less

pronounced, as if there is a difficulty moving the different parts of the body.

*Main activity*

- Start to move as if the movements are painful to make. Start to embody the movements of the Fisher King. Imagine that the movements take you into the wasteland. Move through the wasteland developing the character of the Fisher King.

- On a sheet of paper each person writes the words: 'I am the Fisher King – my land is barren, I am wounded.'

- Continue to write in free-flowing style. Answer the questions:

  (a)   Why are you called the Fisher King?
  (b)   What is happening to your land?
  (c)   How does your wound affect you?
  (d)   What was the land like before it became barren?

- Seated in a circle, experiment with a 'voice' for the King. Share these character sketches with others.

- Each person creates an environment for their King. Using chairs, tables, fabrics and cushions, create the place the King inhabits most frequently. Inhabit the place as the Fisher King. Take time to create a posture and the position that is most comfortable for easing the pain of the wound.

*Closure*

- Moving around the room, de-construct the environments, revitalising the body. Shake, stretch and resume normal gait. Greet other people by name, shake hands, allow the body to become relaxed.

- Go back to sitting in the circle. Is each group member clear about what he or she wants to 'leave' in the group room after the session?

- Goodbyes.

*Purpose: to explore the concept of being wounded and what this means for each person. To explore the effects of the person's perceptions of the environment.*

## Sessions 9 and 10

(The following structures will extend through sessions 9 and 10.)

*Warm-up*

- Greetings.

*Main activity*

- Reconstruct the environment of the Fisher King.

- Form pairs. One person elects to be the Fisher King; the other person is a knight who will eventually ask the King the question, 'What ails thee?' Establish the character of the visitor as someone who is gentle, caring and kind.

- The Fisher King enters the environment constructed for him. Take time to really establish the character. During this time the partner experiments with the knight's movements, voice and characterisations.

- When both partners are ready they start to enact the drama: the first entrance of the visitor, the interactions between the knight and the King, the asking of the question 'What ails thee?' and the response.

- When everyone has played the knight and the King, ask the group to reflect on the drama.

*Closure*

- Reflect on your experience of the session.
- Goodbyes.

## Session 11

*Warm-up*

- Walk around the room with greetings.

*Main activity*

- A healing Grail ritual is constructed for each Fisher King. Each member uses his or her own Grail. (The ritual may be the same as or different from the one created earlier.)
- Reflect on each ritual after it has been 'performed'.

*Closure*

- Reflect on the session. How did it feel to you?
- Goodbyes.

## Session 12

*Warm-up*

- Walk around the room greeting others. Be aware that this is the penultimate session.

*Main activity*

- Reflect on the healing of the King and the effect of the Grail.
- Decide what people will do with their Grails.
- Reflect on the question, 'What ails thee?' What purpose does it have?

*Closure*

- How did the session feel to you?
- Say goodbye, thanking the other people in the group.

*Purpose: to lead gradually on to a sense of completeness with regard to the course of sessions as a unified experience.*

## Session 13

*Warm-up*

- Walk around the room, saying hello for the last time.

*Main activity*

- Consolidation: each person makes everyone else in the group (and themselves) a Grail card (a memento of the drama) and these are distributed round the group.
- Thank-yous and goodbyes.

*Closure*

- Each group member devises a closing ritual as a way of saying a final goodbye to the group.

*Purpose: to provide tangible reminders of the Grail experience for the future.*

*Note:* The Grail Legend may need to be adapted to the cultural backgrounds, contexts and needs of the client group. The characters of the Fisher King and the knight are male and some negotiation will be needed with female participants.

The Grail Legend concerns metaphysical ideas, feelings and values. However, the meaning of our life is also influenced by social and political constraints. Dramatherapy can be a very practical way of encouraging us to take stock of what is actually going on around us in the world.

In the following section we look at an example of the way in which dramatherapy can be used to deal with situations involving social prejudices. This is a 12-week group structure for sessions lasting 1½ hours.

## Session 1

In a seated circle group members exchange names, first in pairs then in the whole group. What kind of group is it going to be? As they talk about the group, people are asked to become aware of the wider implications of culture. They 'brainstorm' what the word means to group members. What do social rules mean to people? Do they help or hinder the way lives are lived? The ideas are put on to a sheet of paper and kept in a safe place until session 2.

## Session 2

*Warm-up*

- Walk around the room, becoming aware of the barriers that exist (walls, furniture, unsafe places). Become aware of boundaries that are created by each person, by moving around other people, finding safe places to walk in, maintaining own body space and staying within own physical capabilities.

- Discuss the difference between boundaries and barriers. What is the difference between a boundary that is created to promote safety and a barrier that seems to limit movement? What body reactions were felt?

*Main activity*

- The large sheet of paper containing the brainstormed words is displayed so group members can refresh their memories from the previous session. Each person has a smaller (A4) sheet of paper and draws a circle in the centre of the page.

- Inside the circle, put words that link with each person's individual concept/experience of culture. This can be as broad as the interpretations agreed at the brainstorming session.

- After about five minutes, group members use the rest of the paper to write words based on the boundaries and barriers that are created by or linked to culture.

- Bring these sheets into the large group and discuss. What are the main issues raised? How do these affect people on a day-to-day basis?

*Closure*

- Form a standing circle.

- First say goodbye to other people in the way that you usually do. Then, one person says 'goodbye' in his or her own way and the others repeat this, taking care to say it in the same way as the 'leader'.

## Session 3

*Warm-up*

- Decide on a particular kind of movement to make with your body. Extend this to involve other parts of the body. (The starting point may be only a slight movement.) Focus on the rhythm of the initial movement, move feet to some rhythm, then knees and so on up the body. Start to move around the room using the same movements.

- Find a partner and look at his or her movements. When ready, start to move around the room copying your partner's movements. Change places.

*Discussion: how did it feel to take on someone else's movements?*

*Main activity*

- Consider times when we are forced to take on someone else's rhythm. This might be a work rhythm, a gender rhythm, a class rhythm or other way of being that is not familiar and feels forced. Start to make a movement that represents or shows this rhythm. Find a partner and show this movement. View your partner's movement.

- Start to extend your own movement. Move away from your partner, move around the room. Become aware of what these movements do to your body.

*Discussion: what effect did these movements have on your body?*

- Each person finds his or her own space in the room. Stand very still. Feel your body frozen by the constraints imposed by having to copy someone. Experience the constraints in each muscle.

- Imagine that your body is surrounded by a cocoon-like substance. Imagine it enclosing you. Move your arm slowly; push against the enclosures of the cocoon. Slowly push the enclosing substance away. Push with your head, then feet, then knees, then hips, then shoulders, then back. Keep pushing as the cocoon gradually starts to give way. Step from the cocoon and stretch, feeling a fresh energy flowing through your body. Move on the spot, then start to move around the room.

*Closure*

- Standing in a circle, one by one each person shows their movements of 'freedom' to others.
- Repeat and say 'goodbye' as you carry on moving.

## Session 4

*Warm-up*

- Walk around the room. Stretch and find ways to release tension and relax your body.
- Make your movements larger, taking up more and more space.
- Form a standing circle. Greet one another while making the 'freedom' movement from session 3.
- Remain in the circle. Each person shows their movement and other group members copy it three times.

*Main activity*

- People return to their own movements. Try to establish the core of your movement. What is the centre of the energy flow?
- Start miming everyday activities at work, in public and at home. Try and contact the centre of the energy found in your own 'freedom' movement.

*Discussion: how did these movements affect the activity?*

- In groups of four or five, discuss social/cultural barriers that stand in the way of achieving the sense of freedom.
- Return to the large group and continue to discuss these issues in terms of barriers and boundaries. Each person considers the social and cultural barriers that prevent her or him reaching the state of freedom. Do this standing up.

- Standing in a circle, experiment with balance. Try to find a position in which your body feels 'grounded'. Focus on the words 'I have the right'. Say them out loud, starting softly and increasing the volume. Move your body to the rhythm of the words.

- Start to move around the room, vocalising 'I have the right'. Say the words as strongly as you can, finding different rhythms for them and expressing them in your body movements.

- Return to the standing circle. In turn, each person goes into the centre of the circle and takes up their posture for 'I have the right'. Then say the words, creating the movement to fit them. Then add 'to _____'. For example, 'I have the right to my opinion', 'I have the right to equality', 'I have the right to walk the streets without being stared at', 'I have the right to justice.'

*Closure*

- Each person confirms the rights of other people in the group.

- Each person says 'goodbye' from a position of power, as if one who knows their right to the position they have claimed.

## Sessions 5, 6 and 7

In these three sessions, each person creates their own drama/piece of theatre about overcoming prejudice and cultural and social oppressions.

*Warm-up*

- Move around the room. Re-focus on the rhythms and movement.

- In a circle, say 'hello' (or other greetings) from your position of power.

*Main activity*

- Share any thoughts that have been present about social or cultural rights.

The following structure is useful (larger groups may divide into smaller ones):

- Each person defines the barriers that prevent them getting their rights. Other group members represent those barriers. They may stand for a particular class, a prejudice, a group of people or a combination of all three. The focus, however, should be on the present (not on any particular episode in your own personal history).
- Boundaries should be defined – no activities which threaten the physical safety of anyone in the group or threats to people outside the group.
- Within this drama the actual social or cultural forces cannot be changed, but the protagonists can experiment with their reactions/responses.

*Closure*

- The drama should finish with the protagonist in their 'freedom' movement. The purpose is to confront the defined social/cultural prejudices.
- Goodbyes.

## Sessions 8, 9 and 10

Along with sessions 11 and 12, these three sessions require some prior experience of drama.

*Warm-up*

- Move around the room, greeting others as you go. Make your movements as free as you can.

*Main activity*

- Group leaders provide newspaper cuttings dealing with the prejudices and social/cultural issues which group members have been addressing. The cuttings are distributed and group members select one each. Time is allowed for people to read the articles.

The following structure is used:

- Each person directs the piece of drama/theatre relating to their chosen article. This can be done in the whole group or by dividing it into two smaller ones. Initially this is a direct, realistic representation of the article.

- In the drama which follows the prejudice is challenged and direct action is shown. This may not alter the social situation, but will illustrate the possibility for change. The most important aspect is to isolate what needs to be changed and what direct action is possible.

- At this point it may be possible to invite other people to view these performances as 'work' in progress.

*Closure*

- People carry out their own 'freedom' movements which are then performed in unison.

- Goodbyes.

## Session 11

*Warm-up*

- Walk around the room, relaxing your body and greeting other people.

*Main activity*

- Look again at the first 'brainstorming' carried out by the group. Discuss any changes that people have made in relation to their own barriers and boundaries.

*Discussion: have people changed or reviewed any of their own prejudices during the group time? What have people learned from each other? What direct action can be taken outside the group? What are the main reasons for prejudice? What thanks do group members want to give each other? Dramatise these thank-yous.*

*Closure*

- Standing in a circle, say goodbyes and express hopes for other group members.

## Session 12

*Warm-up*

- Walk around the room, relaxing your body and greeting one another.

*Main activity*

- Consider the boundaries of culture and how culture can actually provide safe boundaries. What will people use to empower themselves in the future?

*Closure*

- Goodbyes. People reconfirm their hopes for each other.

# CHAPTER 7

# Making Sense of the Past

## Dramatherapy and Story

When we look back over our lives, we tend to see them as a kind of story, with ourselves as the central character. We become very conscious of this when somebody says 'Tell me about yourself' and we find ourselves going over all the things that have happened to us. They may go on to ask what we think was the most important thing in our lives; on the other hand they may not need to enquire about this because we have made it quite clear in our story. They will know without needing to be told what kind of story they are listening to – happy, sad, bitter, ironic, funny or any combination of these – and what are the most important things in it.

Your story reflects your state of mind, not only in the things you are describing but also in the way you are describing them and the order in which you think of them. This is not surprising, of course. If you want your story to be sad, to express the sadness you are feeling, you will tell it in a way that brings your sadness home to people – as, of course, you would if you wanted to make them laugh, or stir them to anger, or get any kind of feeling across at all. You will stress some things and underplay others: you will do things not only by means of the words you choose and your actual tone of voice, but also by the order in which you say them, picking out the parts of the story you want to underline and bring home to whomever is listening.

The point we want to stress is that this is something everyone does quite naturally. It is the way we communicate with one another, particularly the way we talk about ourselves. We tell each other stories to give each other meaning. Strictly speaking, we tell our story to ourselves, rehearsing and rearranging it in our own mind before offering it to someone else, who accepts it and makes it real for us. They make it real for us by accepting it from us. You could say our stories exist *between*. This is why being a member of a group of people who are exchanging stories is such a rewarding experience, as everybody feels strengthened in themselves by having their personal stories rectified as genuinely theirs.

This process of realising your story is an ongoing one. We do it in our own minds, holding silent conversations with ourselves, between the various selves we can imagine being. If we cannot put any kind of story together which seems to make sense to us – sense about ourselves – we are confused and restless. People in this state of mind feel empty. The world lacks meaning. Nothing 'fits'. However much we arrange and rearrange the things that are happening and have happened to us, no story even begins to emerge. Not even a tragic one, although this kind of meaninglessness is perhaps the worst tragedy of all. We have the building blocks – everything we go through provides us with a supply of these – but cannot build ourselves a house to live in. This is where dramatherapy is so much help.

Dramatherapy helps us rearrange our stories as a way of reordering our lives. As we said above, our story represents the way we regard *ourselves*. There is no final version of ourselves, no fixed scale of importance attached to the various things that have happened to us in life which determines the way we arrange our material, the order in which we place the various episodes within our personal saga. Sometimes we fall victim to the vivid and convincing dramas we create about and for ourselves. People can quite easily become hypnotised by stories which they themselves have constructed, convinced by the strength of their feelings and their own dramatic sense that this is the only possible account any one could give of them. Dramatherapy encourages us to be flexible and adaptive in our storytelling; if we seem somehow to have lost our story altogether, dramatherapy helps us set about finding one.

One of the most powerful ways that dramatherapy works is by creating *the story of the group*. This story is made up of all the personal histories of those who belong to it. In dramatherapy we take these stories and expand them by relating them all to a wider and more comprehensive 'group story', one that is able to feed itself back into each individual's past experience and give that person courage and inspiration as they look back on things done and said, the people they felt able to be and actually *were* in that special place and time.

Dramatherapy uses story to heal stories. The life of the group becomes a story in itself in order to speak the language of ongoing human experience, which is, in fact, story-language. Certainly this group life would create its own history – all human groups do this. Dramatherapy, however, uses dramatic structure to transform this narrative raw material into a powerful episode in the lives of the members of the group. These lives are able to stand together as a connected event. We are able to give them a definite shape in order to make a kind of message from them, a message about life that we can learn something from. This kind of thing rarely happens in the flux of experiences that constitute what we call ordinary life – but when it does we make good use of it, judging everything else that happens by the standard it sets, and allowing it to stand as a sign of hope for us, that life *can* have shape and meaning.

This is the hope we use to live by. If stories increase this hope they are necessary for maintaining life. To put this another way: we know we are alive as people when we can give our lives shape by dramatising them in this way, because the more we can see ourselves as living out a story which appears to us to have some kind of point to it, the more point we ourselves have as people. This, of course, is Moreno's (1977) purpose in enabling people to become protagonists of their own psychodramas. As William Saroyan (1996) puts it in *The Time of Your Life*, 'it takes a lot of rehearsing for a man to get to be himself'. This kind of rehearsing is vitally important for our growth as human beings. We all need it, not only people whose sense of identity is or has become exceptionally frail. It has been said that 'to become a self is to appropriate a past' (Crites 1986, p.164). This is because it is only in the light of the past, of what we have been, that we can change and take on a future which is personal to us – 'only a self can amend itself'.

But we cannot do this alone. Our story depends on other people's stories. Stories must be shared, because in order to form genuine human relationships there must always be some kind of common ground. A shared story is the basis of a shared relationship. We do not have to have the same story – which would be impossible – or even one which is recognisably similar to someone else's. The way that stories meet is through mutual recognition – the presence of things in your story that remind me of things in mine. These 'interior correspondences' are the elements in other people's stories which we find so valuable when we are engaged in working on our own personal narrative. Things that never really happened to us at all are *built into* things that certainly did by a psychological process which can make other people's experiences 'grist to our mill' as they help us to reorganise our past by re-creating their own stories with our assistance. When this process is consciously undertaken and we set out to put together a kind of corporate story that will somehow involve elements of everybody's individual, personal histories and synthesise them with or in a new story, one specially created by us to reproduce no one's actual history while referring in a personal way to everyone's, then we have begun to do dramatherapy.

At this level of experience, story and drama are the same thing. No record of events can really be called a story in this archetypal sense unless it comes across in this dramatic way, as something both *recognisable* and *new*. They are new because we have just created them in this new form. They are recognisable because we are used to this way of making sense of things – or at least, trying to do so. The process of making recognisable stories is very familiar to us, unconsciously at least. As we said, this is the way we try to make life coherent. Stories, dramatic stories, are powerful symbols of completeness. As such, they have a beginning, a middle and an end. (Euclid, the inventor of geometry, is traditionally believed to have referred to the number 3 as 'the number of perfection'.) It is a completeness which contains movement, however. In other words, stories are the symbols of, or signs for, perfect processes. Stories progress and communicate the idea of progression to us who listen to them – even more so if we involve ourselves bodily by acting them out. As the story moves, we move with it.

The movement embodied in stories and dramas is quite straight-forward. We imagine ourselves (along with our companions) moving from one point in time to another. The point is, however, that for the process to work properly we have to imagine it in the right way; that is, in the way movement is thought about or communicated by story. This is not the way we tend to regard movement. Story is based on the way *people* move, rather than the movement of things; or rather, it is constructed to take account of movement that involves states of mind and soul – what we call experimental or life-movement.

Movement like this always takes up more time and space than we habitually expect it to do – or plan for. This is because it involves an extra stage in the actual process of change. Life-movement involves a middle stage, a time when the old state of affairs is over but the new one has not yet begun. In other words, stories about people always move from A to C via B. This basic framework may be subdivided, however, and the structure of most stories is considerably more subtle than this. The point is, however, that however complicated a story may be it still remains an event which takes place in three stages, a balanced work of art.

Stories are balanced round whatever happens in Stage B, the middle stage. For a story to exist as a story, it must have a climax of some kind. This is very important and the value of the climax, its dramatic impact, tends to govern the way we rate the entire story. If this thing – whatever it is – had not happened, there would be no story to tell; if it had not happened *like that*, it would not have been half so good a story. This is the climax of the plot. Stage A is obviously very important as well, because stories have to start off in a definite way, firmly rooted in some kind of recognisable landscape, a reality with which the audience (those to whom the story is addressed) is familiar, so that we can 'start off from where we are'. This need not be where we actually are, of course. Many wonderful stories start off in some kind of mythical past or hypothetical future and run their entire course without leaving the framework they have established at the beginning, *once upon a time* – but it must be a time and place that we can imagine here and now, and preferably one we have often been to before, one way or another, that is. Stage C is the story's destination, our point of arrival – so this is obviously just as important otherwise there would be no point in setting out on our imaginative journey in the first place. In Stage C we come home, so this must be recognisable too; only this has to be recognisably *different*, so that we can feel that the story has added something to our experience, so that we are not exactly the same as we were before we heard it. In some way, by engaging our imagination, it has expanded us.

Stages A, B and C are always present in any story. They do not necessarily have to follow each other in this story. Part of a storyteller's skill lies in juggling with the succession of events and situations within the tale that is being told – hence the use of stories-within-stories and plays-within-plays, and the even more common dependence on flashbacks to keep the audience guessing. All the same, at whatever point in the performance they may actually occur, there is always a beginning, a middle and an end, an underlying 'shape of the story' to bring its message home to us.

Although stories stay the same basic shape, they certainly differ from one another in *size*. Some are very big, very important, indeed. The theme of some stories is nothing less than the transformation of the world and everything in it. Such mega-stories may be religious; they may also be political, cultural, scientific. Whatever they are, they reflect the storyteller's commitment to a particular and well-defined philosophy of what life itself is actually about. Life and death, in fact. They do not simply reflect this, they embody it, using our natural ability to identify our own experience with the living and dying of 'the people in the story' so that we share in their adventures and make them our own. These are stories that carry weight for us. By existing and requiring such a degree of commitment, they give significance to storytelling itself.

Dramatherapy has its own way of telling stories. A better way of saying this would be to say that there is a particular dramatherapy approach to story, the aim of which is to find a way of letting the story tell *itself* through the feelings, ideas and actions of the people in the group. They do not need to come along to the session already prepared to tell stories, or even to take part in a dramatised story which the dramatherapist has chosen for them. This can happen, but it certainly does not have to. The most characteristic dramatherapy approach is for a story to emerge from the group itself, as it did in the examples given in Chapter 6. This may or may not be a story that already exists (like *Sleeping Beauty*); or it may be one that the group has invented for itself (as in the 'social justice' example). The important thing to grasp is that both kinds of stories resemble each other so far as their basic shape is concerned. Because both stories are about change and both embody a process of change, both have the same underlying order of events.

Dramatherapy aims at encouraging positive changes within human experience. It is rooted in the understanding that drama and story are themselves *about change*. Whether its raw material is simply a record of ordinary events that someone has 'made into a story' or a profoundly tragic or comic fable belonging to the cultural heritage of men and women throughout the world, it will always constitute an image of transformation. The shape of what happens here remains the same. Whether the subject matter is ordinary or fantastic, trivial or profound, the experience is one of movement. *The shape is shared* and because of this, even our hastily patched together sagas remind us of changes that are of infinitely greater significance – the vital life and death transformations put into fictional form so that they resonate down the ages. These are stories that are never entirely forgotten because they emerge in different versions wherever human beings meet to tell each other tales and ponder about life's underlying meaning. Because the meaning we give to and find in life is itself a story about changes, such stories can never be forgotten.

The underlying shape of story and drama is A–B–C – a beginning, a middle and an end. This provides a framework for a succession of episodes, some of which resemble stories in themselves because they, too, are accounts of the way particular problems are solved and difficulties overcome – problems and difficulties that must be dealt with 'on the way to' surmounting the story's central, climactic obstacle, the one that by being surmounted will really constitute change.

Stories can be any length, so long as they narrate some kind of action that we can recognise as complete in itself – a kind of event made up of various things that belong to the story which altogether add up to a real conclusion, a recognisable change in the state of affairs. What these ingredients actually are, of course, depends on the particular story being told. On the other hand, they do fit into certain very definite categories, dealing first of all with *plot* (the things that happen) and second with *setting* (when and where they happen). Plot elements are crucial to the story in itself, the story *as a story*; but no amount of dramatic impact or dramatic irony will help us relate to the story so that we can share its own particular world, if we have no way of finding out where that world is. In other words, if we are unable to locate it with regard to our own experience, whether this is actual or imaginary. Stories have to comfort and surprise us at the same time: nobody knows this better than a dramatherapist. One of the ways they are able to do this is by means of the familiarity of their general structure.

For instance: to begin with, attention is paid to the place where the story is set and the people whom it concerns (particularly the hero or heroine). 'Once upon a time, in a high castle in a low valley, there lived a king and queen. They had a daughter whom they loved. She, however, was a restless and adventurous girl and...' In other words, there are three principal elements in this first section: *landscape, dwelling* and *character*. At this point, before the story has begun to move at all, we hear of the first opportunity for movement – the first *difficulty*. This does not arrive as a total surprise, the scene already being set for trouble by the foregoing information about character. (This is an adventurous princess; we are expecting her to run into difficulties. We identify with her but cannot help feeling a little apprehensive.) This first difficulty or set of difficult circumstances calls forth some help for the princess in the shape of another character, either a *friend* or an *enemy*, who is either a companion (there is always a source of support somewhere, although it may sometimes seem a bit out of the ordinary) or a thorn-in-the-flesh. This is the relationship which, in one way or another, for better or worse, makes the story real – an ongoing theme of a personal kind which holds the structure together. Having established this, the story moves into its central section, what might be called the journey itself. (This is the 'transforming action' of the story and consists of a series of trials or tests which must be endured and overcome by the hero or heroine.) In many legends, folk tales and myths this part contains a succession of *three problems*, each of which seems impossible to solve. One after another, all three must be solved before the heroine or hero can move onwards to the third stage in the story, which she typically does on her own, having sadly parted company with her friend, or finally rid herself of her enemy (or both) after the solution of the final, crucial problem.

These problems are more than ordinary domestic difficulties, of course. They are meant to stand for the most intractable of all human situations. They are 'all the dangers and disasters of life rolled into one'. Metaphorically speaking, they are often death itself. In the story they and everything they stand for has been challenged head-on and finally and utterly defeated. The conclusion of the story establishes a complete state of affairs. This is the celebrated 'transformation scene' (the scene when everything has been transformed. As we saw, the business of transforming it was not nearly so clear-cut and serene.) One way or another this is always a homecoming. In some stories, when victory at the second stage has been secured only by the death of the central character, this final section may be a funeral; in many cases it is a wedding. Whatever its actual subject matter, it is always a definite statement, the final period to a sentence. Consequently the heroine or hero does not have to return to the place from which she or he first set out. In some ways it is better if they do not do this, because the story is really about change. If we have solved problems like these, passed through a time like that, wherever we arrive will be home to us. Those stories, legends and myths which involve the death of the hero or heroine carry reconciliation beyond the grave.

The overall shape of stories like these is as follows:

A   *The introduction*

   Landscape – Dwelling – Characters

B   *The action*

   (a)   Difficulty – Friend or enemy (or both)
   (b)   Three problems (in ascending order of difficulty)
       (i)   Problem I
       (ii)  Problem II
       (iii) Problem III
   (c)   Three solutions (each accompanying one of the problems)
       (i)   Solution I
       (ii)  Solution II
       (iii) Solution III

C   *The conclusion*

   Being a single, final statement (the complement/answer to part A), part C has only one section.

Put like this, it is easy to see how the story falls into three parts, and how the middle part is itself divided into three sections, corresponding to the three problems. The most important problem is the third one. This preserves the dynamism needed to carry the tale onwards to its final conclusion.

Individual people within a group have their own stories. These are expanding in scope and developing in clarity – developing as stories – day by day, minute by minute. Simply being in the group affects the individual stories. The group, too, has its corporate story, its self-narrative as a group of people that shares certain experiences and forms certain relationships which belong to its life together as a group. These two dimensions – the group and the individual – are, of course, inseparable in our actual experience of a particular situation. The best way of describing the quality of life they represent would be to speak of 'the life of the group' – that is, the life we exchange with the individual members of the group, the group itself, and ourselves apart from the group. It is this subject matter, this narrative material, that we use to create the stories which express and heal us. The life of the group is all these histories – expanded, deepened, enriched by sharing and focusing.

The means of focusing all this potential may be a story borrowed from somewhere else (folklore, mythology, history, literature etc.). The story is taken over because it resonates so powerfully and expressively with the group's own story, and because it already possesses the shape we are searching for in our own lives: the shape of the story. In taking it over we transform it and are imaginatively transformed by it. In other words, the shape of our own world, our own *story*, is changed. To use story like this is to allow it to affect the way we live with ourselves and one another.

To have this effect, stories must be properly told. In this, skill is important but not essential; much superb storytelling is as instinctive as the search for meaning. Love, however, is essential. When a group becomes involved in a story so that it begins to share imaginative being in and with the story, it begins to love. The act of shared narration leads individuals and groups out from where they are, out from themselves to meet the Other.

Stories are about meeting and sharing – meeting to share. Alida Gersie and Nancy King (1990) state the principle as it is expressed in the fundamental act of 'telling a story':

> Each story is re-created in the interaction between teller and listener. It is their relationship which causes a story to come to life. The ebb and flow of the listener's concentration and attention influence its dynamics. The relationship between teller and listener is always intimate. The closeness is generated by the interconnection between the one who tells and the one who listens. By the act of sharing highly individual or collective, symbolic material with another to whom this same symbolic structure matters, a special, fragile bond is created which lasts for as long as the story is allowed to continue. (Gersie and King 1990, p.32)

Dramatherapy often provides the setting for individual people to tell stories, either to one another or the group. In dramatherapy, however, the setting *is* the story. Here we tell each other our own story by creating a shared history.

## Karen: A case study

*Karen is 44. She has a history of depressive episodes since the age of 34. Major manifestations of depressions include low mood, inability to concentrate, lack of self-esteem, anhedonia, despair. After assessment and history-taking, the initial sessions of work revealed an image of depression as a large tunnel which goes on for ever, with no light at the end.*

### *Creating the environment (the set)*

EXTENSION OF IMAGE

It is a dark tunnel, covered in lichen and moss. Water drips from the walls, making a dull, frightening sound. It is deep in the ground. The walls are of concrete.

*This picture is extended by client and therapist to include some more hopeful elements.*

Above the tunnel, which is very deep in the ground, is a green field. Children play there and in spring a maypole is erected. People celebrate the coming of May. May brings flowers and brightness.

PROJECTION OF IMAGE

Karen creates a small picture on an A4 sheet of paper. There is a long tunnel at the bottom of the page. It stretches from edge to edge, creating a continuous line. At the top of the page is a thin green line with two yellow flowers which touch the top edge of the paper.

EXTENSION OF DRAWN IMAGE BY FOCUSING ON THE SPACE
BETWEEN THE TUNNEL AND THE FIELD

Karen completes the image by drawing the roots from the flowers. These run from the stems halfway down the page. She adds some roots from the grass which is represented by the green line. These are longer than the flower roots and nearly reach the tunnel. Using a light brown pencil she makes lines to represent the earth. More pressure is applied near the tunnel and the lines are heavier and darker. Finally she uses a blue crayon to represent the rain water that nourishes the roots and maintains growth.

*The purpose is to find representations of her inner strengths. These are represented by the roots and the water that promotes growth. The therapist prompts by focusing on spaces and asking open questions about the grass and flowers and how they survive. No interpretations are made of the images she creates.*

### Inhabiting the image

Karen is asked to list the objects represented in the picture. Her list is: ROOTS, FLOWERS, EARTH, WATER, THICK WALLS, SPACES. Under each word she adds those that she connects with the top word.

| ROOTS | FLOWERS | EARTH | WATER | THICK WALLS | SPACES |
|-------|---------|-------|-------|-------------|--------|
| Firm | Blooming | Moist | Fluid | Solid | Empty |
| Sturdy | Fresh | Solid | Life-giving | Closed | Void |
| Supporting | Bright | Rich | Flowering | Old | Distant |
| Connected | Connected | | | Impene-trable | Resisting |

These words are used in order to form the basis of a script. Karen puts her finger on one of the objects she has listed and speaks as the object. She speaks slowly, hesitantly and with eyes downcast. At one point she stops and says she feels silly. Her attention is diverted back to the image and she is reassured that there are no right sentences to form and that this is just a different way of expressing her feelings.

Her script is:

*ROOTS: We are strong and supportive. We grow slowly but surely. We connect the earth with the air and the rain. We grow at an even pace and support the living plant. We are hidden but vital. Without us nothing can survive. Grass roots need to be longer than flower roots because grass is common, taken for granted and crushed underfoot. (Very long pause.) We are important. We are hidden but strong and sturdy.*

*FLOWERS: We like the sun, we are open and bright. People like us. We indicate that it is summer and a time to be in the sun.*

*EARTH: I am moist and nourishing. I am a rich mixture of elements. I hold the rain and allow the roots to flourish. I am solid and provide a strong foundation for all of the things above.*

*WATER: Sometimes people don't want me when I fall as rain, but I am essential to life. I keep the roots, flowers and earth together to help them to grow and produce life. I am soft and giving.*

*THICK WALLS: I protect. I keep people away. I am very, very strong and solid. I have been here for many, many years and I cannot be penetrated or demolished. I protect. I will not allow those from either side of me to meet.*

*SPACES: We resist. We are empty. We do not want to be intruded upon. We resist any attempt to fill us. We are voids that like to remain distant from any interactions with others. We are alone and want to select how we are. We do not want to make contact with the living things around us until we are ready.*

*The purpose here is to allow each object in the environment to express a view and so contribute its perspective on its place within the completed picture – so as to extend the metaphor of tunnel and field.*

### Creating characters

Karen is asked to introduce characters. She chooses people, but the characters could be animals, supernatural beings or objects. Through a process of negotiation she decides on two characters – the person in the tunnel and the person in the field. She writes a short character analysis on each person:

*MARIA (the person in the field)*

*I am 78 and I have spent my life in the country. I enjoy the fresh air and the freedom to walk across the fields and in the lanes and woods. I live in a small cottage on the outskirts of a small village. I am content and create my own routines for a satisfying life.*

*I have always lived in the country. As a child I was able to roam freely and the animals were my friends. I particularly loved the rabbits and the small animals that lived in the fields and near the streams. As I grew up I realised that I did not want to move to a town or city. As a child I played with some children from the village school but mainly enjoyed my own company, creating stories about the animals and the woods. When I was a teenager I became even more independent and spent my time without the company of other people of my own age. My interest in country crafts developed and I started to become interested in pottery based on Celtic design. This interest became my living later in life. I developed a very small business with my pottery and made a comfortable living. As I look back I do feel that I made the right choices.*

*DELIA (the person in the tunnel)*

*I am 22 (I think). It is difficult to recall a life before the time in the tunnel. I hate it here. I can only sit in an uncomfortable position. I ache and ache. My back and limbs are cramped and I cannot move. The noise of the water dripping drives me mad. The constant noise echoes through the tunnel and I wait for the next drop to fall. It is wet and dark. I feel frozen but I can't move. I don't know how I got here.*

*I know there is life above me but I feel disconnected from it. I think but I capture the thoughts. I do not know day from night, I have no concept of time. I am here. I do not have any connection with past or future. I don't know where I came from or where I can go. I am stuck. I am not aware of anything except the darkness and the damp. I do not have the strength to scream or to call for help.*

THERAPIST'S THOUGHTS AND REFLECTIONS

Karen has created two solitary characters with different outlooks and philosophies on life. There are several options that can be followed up:

1    To focus on Delia and to create her life before the tunnel. Although she has stated she cannot recall this time it would be possible for Karen to take on the role of writer or narrator to recall the time the character cannot recall.

2    To develop the roles of the objects in the environment in order to solicit their views on the person in the tunnel. How can they help?

3    To focus on Maria as a potential helper/healer-through-experience.

4    To develop the opportunities provided by Maria's childhood experiences of creating stories.

*Karen as storyteller*

Perhaps Karen can expand on her own images of healing through the metaphor of her story.

The option of Maria's childhood stories offers potential for assimilating many of the images created so far and provides distance for expanding the symbolic range. It was this method that the client chose.

*MARIA'S STORIES*

*1 The Rabbit Who Liked to Eat Carrots*

*Once upon a time there was a young rabbit who had just left home. He said goodbye to his parents one sunny day at the end of spring. The flowers were bright and colourful. He was sad to leave his childhood home but also very excited about going into the world to have adventures. His mother had warned him about the dangers that foxes and other creatures of the night could present to him but he was sure he could look after himself. He was a confident rabbit with his mind set on finding lots of carrots to eat. The one thing he loved to do was to eat carrots. A short distance away he came across a huge house with an equally huge garden. All this meant to him was a place where carrots could grow. He rushed into the garden and then rushed around looking for the carrot patch. As he rushed he ignored everything else in the garden and forgot about danger. At last he found the carrots. He stopped and looked in amazement. There were rows and rows of carrots. He sniffed in the wonderful aroma. He feasted his eyes on the sight of the green vegetation with the promise of the delicious orange food waiting to be munched. He started to dig for the carrots. As he uprooted the heavenly vegetables he nibbled and chewed until he was full.*

*For weeks, indeed months, he stayed in the garden eating carrots and then sleeping. He did not create a rabbit hole but slept under the cover of a huge dock leaf. As time went by he became fatter and fatter until he was hardly able to move. Still he ate carrots and he slept. One day it was quite cold and he wanted to build a place to live, but he did not want to dedicate much time to this as it would have interrupted his carrot eating. He made a half-hearted attempt to dig a hole but soon gave up and returned to eating carrots. He was completely unaware that he was in danger. The gardener was becoming increasingly annoyed about the loss of his produce and the accompanying mess. He had decided to set a trap. Some of the frogs in a nearby pond watched him and decided to tell the rabbit. They waited until the gardener had gone home and told the rabbit about the danger he was in. The rabbit didn't know what to do. He didn't want to leave the garden, but he didn't have a hiding place. The frogs told him about a hole in the wall where he could dig quickly. The rabbit dug the hole near the wall and hid. The hole was warm and comfortable and he was safe. He lived in the garden for the rest of his life. The frogs always warned him about the gardener and he only ate enough carrots to prevent hunger. He was happy.*

2 *The Wicked Forest*

*In the dim and distant past there once stood a huge forest. It was dark in the forest. The sun was never able to penetrate the trees so the undergrowth was moss and other dark tangles of things that grew close to the ground. Snakes, spiders and rats lived in the middle of the trees. In the centre was a huge pond with stagnant water. Water snakes, toads and huge eels lived in the pond.*

*One day a young field mouse was playing at being a brave adventurer. He strayed further and further away from the field. He came nearer and nearer to the forest. He became aware of the darkness of the shadow, but told himself that he was a brave adventurer and had to continue his journey. Eventually he found himself deep in the forest. He was very frightened. Very, very frightened. He carried on into the forest and it became darker and darker. He reached a stagnant pond. It was horrible. It stank. He sat and cried until he couldn't cry any more. He became still and stayed so still he couldn't move. He was so scared.*

*After a long, long time he heard a soft noise. He became more frightened. The noise became louder. He couldn't look. It was a tiny bird who had come to help him. 'Follow me,' said the bird. 'No,' said the mouse. The bird and the mouse stayed together in silence for weeks. Eventually the mouse looked at the bird. For weeks he looked. After 6 months the mouse moved. The bird moved too. After a year the mouse let the bird lead him out of the forest.*

*When the mouse reached the edge of the forest he saw that the bird had bright, beautiful colours. The mouse said 'Thank you' and the bird sang brightly and then went back into the forest to help other frightened creatures.*

Karen becomes tearful while creating these stories. The main connections she makes with her life were the pattern of overreaching, being foolish and not making provision for 'things that might happen', being immobilised by fear of the unknown and finding help difficult to accept. She has been able to express many of her fears through the metaphors of the stories, and says she would like to know more about the child who had created them.

She and the therapist re-read the character sketch she has written for Maria, and she adds a description of Maria's childhood, saying that she was a kind, thoughtful child. The therapist asks how she would react/feel if she was aware of Delia's plight in the tunnel? Karen considers this for some time and eventually states that she would want to help by telling her the stories.

*The dramatic method that they choose is to create a puppet to represent Delia in the tunnel and for Karen to play the character of Maria as a child.*

PREPARATION

Karen makes a 12-inch hand/glove puppet from tights and fabrics. She selects dark, thick material for her dress and black wool for her hair. A tunnel is made from cardboard and crêpe paper. This is then cut in half lengthways, to allow the puppet to be seen. Karen spends some time positioning the puppet. She and the therapist rehearse the character of 'Maria the child', trying out different ways of speaking and moving in role.

*Between sessions Karen has written the stories in a brightly coloured notebook and added some illustrations. She reports that she has been able to concentrate on this task and has enjoyed the process. Now she is ready to work with the puppets.*

### *The dramatic action 1*

The Delia puppet is placed in the tunnel which is itself located under a table (the darkest place in the room). Karen sits cross-legged on the floor and 'inhabits' the character of Maria aged 7. She allows herself time to connect with the breathing and voice of the characters and finds the right way to hold the notebook. In a friendly manner, she reads the two stories to Delia.

After she has done this, Karen spends a little time de-roling from Maria. The therapist encourages her to explore the positive aspects of the child she has been playing. She herself comments on some of the things that have helped her:

- the breathing patterns that enabled her body to feel refreshed
- the posture which 'freed a fresh energy'
- the sheer enjoyment of telling the stories.

The next stage is to work with the Delia puppet. Karen is able to enter the space under the table. She holds the puppet and strokes her hair, then the fabric of her dress. Asked to describe her actions, she states that the puppet looks dejected and she is comforting her. She eventually places the puppet over her right hand and puts her back in the tunnel. She continues to stroke her with her left hand, and starts to hum.

Client and therapist work together with the Delia puppet, giving her small movements and a voice. A scenario about Delia's time in the tunnel is developed. She says that she heard the stories, but found it difficult to accept that anyone should spend time telling them to her.

*Throughout the following sessions the therapy is developed through the projections created by the two characters.*

First of all, Delia explores her situation in the tunnel through the continued use of story-making. The therapist reminds Karen of the drawing she had created at the beginning of the therapy. Karen and the therapist discuss how Delia can be made aware of the roots, flowers, earth, water and the spaces that exist beyond the thick walls of the tunnel. Karen eventually decides that the child, Maria, could tell her.

Karen takes time to re-create the character of Maria. She shows Maria the picture and explains the significance of each object. Next, she de-roles and takes up the Delia puppet again. The puppet remembers that she has previously stated that she 'knew there was a life above me'. She ponders on how she can connect with it. She decides that she, too, will create a story.

*DELIA'S STORY (abridged)*

*It was a day in winter. Snow was falling. It was thick snow. It snowed and snowed until the whole earth was covered in a thick blanket of snow. The ponds were frozen and the streams stopped running. Under the ground the roots were storing the moisture from the earth. The larger roots looked after the smaller roots, making sure that they were warm and able to survive the cold winter. The earth around the roots remained moist, it retained its warmth and was able to look forward to the summer.*

*The roots moved cautiously around the spaces. Eventually they were able to surround them in a gentle manner. The edges of the spaces became warm. The snow eventually melted and the earth became more moist. It was able to provide even more nourishment for the roots.*

*The roots grew and started to prepare for the spring when the flowers would grow. They grew downwards too. Eventually they reached the wall of the tunnel. They spread along the width of the wall and looked for cracks they could penetrate. All the time the roots were nourished by the water and they knew that even though they were in a dark place the flowers they would grow would be bright and bask in the sunlight.*

*One day the roots reached the end of the tunnel. It was covered by a thick web that spiders had spun over the centuries. The webs were no longer used by the spiders. The roots slowly broke through the webs and sunlight entered the tunnel. The roots were surprised to note that they had been growing upwards along the tunnel wall. They, too, enjoyed the sun and looking at the flowers and grass they had been supporting.*

*The sunlight flowed gently down the tunnel. It was a long time before the moisture could be cleared.*

The therapist has worked with Karen to create this story by reminding her of the word associations she made with the objects, and helping her brainstorm when she was stuck. The purpose was to extend the metaphors she used to express her feelings of depression at the start of the therapy and to give reality to the contrast between 'light' and 'darkness'.

### The dramatic action 2

Client and therapist return to the puppet. The set is re-created and the puppet, activated by Karen, talks about the sun coming down the tunnel.

'I can feel the warmth, it is good. I can feel the sunlight on my face and shoulders. I want to move. My joints are stiff, I have been here so long. I want to move into the light.'

The next sessions are spent on moving the puppet. She moves very slowly within the cramped conditions of the tunnel. She is eventually able to lie on her front with her face upturned towards the light. Very slowly she moves towards the end of the tunnel, but says she is too frightened to go any further.

*The puppet is expressing Karen's fear. She wants to move forward but feels stuck.*

The therapist suggests that the character of Maria could offer support. Karen agrees. She re-creates this character, sitting on cushions near the end of the tunnel.

As Maria, Karen says, 'It is lonely out here. It is not always sunny. Sometimes it rains; sometimes the wind blows. The light is not blinding. We rest at night and prepare for the day.'

*The therapist notices that Karen is changing her voice while playing Maria. The voice is deeper with more resonance. Karen responds by stating that Maria is growing up. The therapist suggests that the adult Maria is created.*

Some time is spent creating the character of the adult Maria. She sits on a chair rather than cushions. Then she speaks, 'I am here for you. I am here and cannot pull you out of the tunnel. I would like to support you and for you to share my world. I am waiting for you. I can soothe your aching shoulders and tend your hurt.'

Karen asks the therapist to transfer the Delia puppet on to Maria's lap. They discuss ways in which Karen herself can activate the puppet and talk about what Maria's lap might feel like. Karen says it will be soft and welcoming. The therapist brings up the subject of the kind of clothes Maria would wear, and some fabric is selected to represent her dress. The fabric is spread over a cushion on the chair. Karen then activates the puppet, who moves slowly from the tunnel on to the fabric.

*It is important that Karen herself moves the puppet (which represents her depressed self) on to Maria (who represents her healing self). The task of the therapist is to find a dramatic method to enable her to do this in order to allow the process of integration to continue.*

Karen moves on to the chair and re-creates the adult Maria character. She spreads the dress fabric across her legs and puts the puppet on to her lap. She spends about a quarter of an hour stroking the puppet, massaging its shoulders and making soothing noises.

*The comforting of Delia by Maria continues for several sessions.*

The therapist asks Karen about the future of the tunnel. Karen decides that it should be rebuilt. The tunnel is re-made by the addition of cardboard, tissue paper and crêpe paper. It becomes a safe, solid structure with flowers growing at the entrance. Karen states that it is a safe place for people to enter when they want to rest. People can enter and leave at will and the walls will protect them. The Delia puppet is placed on the dress fabric to 'watch' the reconstruction of the tunnel.

*During the closing sessions the functions of the tunnel as a place of safety are confirmed.*

### Consolidation

The therapy is consolidated over the next six sessions by reflecting on the stories, the characters and the environment. What has each of these contributed to the healing process?

Karen takes home the fabric puppet and the new tunnel to remind herself of the journey.

### To sum up

During these sessions, the role of the therapist has been to marry together the creative process and the client's descriptions of her feelings. At the assessment session, Karen supplied a list of negative words which described her body and her feelings. With the therapist she also created a list of opposing words. For example, she felt stuck, heavy, sad and forlorn. These were written thus:

Sad

Forlorn

Stuck

Heavy

Then words that meant the opposite (or more or less so) were added:

Sad       Happy

Forlorn   Content

Stuck     Freed

Heavy     Moving

The list contained 30 words with 30 'opposites'.

Each week both client and therapist examined the list and ticked the appropriate words. By the end of the 40 sessions it showed a significant shift in her perceptions of the way she was feeling. At some point or other, every positive word had been ticked. The therapist noted that there was also a link between the emotions that Karen had experienced in her life between sessions, and the feelings she associated with Delia and Maria.

# CHAPTER 8

# Bringing Words to Life
## Dramatherapy and Text

This is a chapter that almost writes itself. It is about the immense riches stored up in all kinds of written texts. Poems, novels and, of course, plays themselves are an immense storehouse of meaning of the most personal kind. A poem is crystallised personal truth and this is expanded in novels, where the truth takes story form (as, of course, it does in some poems, too). Plays let us clothe these stories, this truth about ourselves with real human flesh and blood. Some plays are like acted poems: *Macbeth, Three Sisters, The Importance of Being Earnest, Waiting for Godot* – all different kinds of acted poetry. Poems, too, come in various sizes, from *The Rime of the Ancient Mariner* to a Japanese haiku. Novels tend to be a bit long, but they all contain situations and relationships that can be acted. In fact, there is an endless choice of material available. It does not even need to seem to be particularly dramatic. Acting makes it into drama. Taking on roles, imagining a situation involving people within particular circumstances, a particular situation, always makes a play. Even when it is a very dull idea, something that seems boring when you read about it, acting brings it to life. Any old situation, so long as it involves people or has parts in it that people can play, will start to seem interesting once you treat it as if it is really happening and happening to *you*. When you use your imagination and play something for real, you bring your own magic.

But there is no reason why you should not decide on something you like – something you yourself find interesting or even inspiring. The point we are making here is simply that there is much more scope for making drama than you might think, and that it is letting yourself get imaginatively involved which makes all the difference. The best results come, of course, when everybody decides to work on a text that they are all interested in or stimulated by; then it can be really exciting, because working with a text lets people relax into what they are doing in a way that other ways of doing drama do not, and this can be an advantage from some points of view. There are at least two ways in which using a written text gives people the confidence to take part in something which would terrify them if they were asked to do it in any other way – if, for instance, they were told to go ahead and make something up for themselves, improvise a scene from their own lives or imitate something they had seen on television. You do not have to get up in a poem or story. You can simply sit and read it. If you have got the courage – or the cheek – you can try reading it aloud, and if other people join in, you have got a play. And the same thing is obviously true about acted plays. Sitting down, reading them, or standing up holding the text in your hands, you are acting and not acting, taking part and observing at the same time. It is as if the words you are reading both lead you into the action of the drama and protect you from some of its impact. In fact, you may very well need protecting, not only from your own nervousness but from the naked force of an author's imagination. Some of the poems, plays and novels that mean most to us do so because the things they are describing are so charged with emotional power – not only for them but for us as well. Fiction often deals in archetypes, symbolic characters and situations that sum up human experience and point beyond it as well – this is what life is like, they say, *your* life too; it is your story as well as theirs.

Sometimes when you come across symbolism like this you are glad you have got a book in your hands. You need something to help you stay with what is being said, what the author is involving you in. What you want to be involved in, if you can only find the courage to cope with it. The book in your hands, or the text on the table in front of you, gives you this courage. It is what we said earlier: some things about us, the things that are most important from an emotional point of view, resist being confronted head-on. The text is a kind of mask. We need it to hide behind.

That is one way of putting it. You might also say that it is a bridge, a link, a source of communication or even revelation. Like theatre itself, it actually reveals things by protecting us from them. Donald Winnicott (1971) talks about the way in which works of art are 'transitional objects', artificial things that we – or somebody – have made up, which have a comforting kind of solidity and allow themselves to be 'pinned down' or, in this case, held in our hands and read by us, either silently to ourselves or aloud with other people. Transitional objects allow us to feel and say things which we would otherwise find difficulty in saying and perhaps even feeling. They are communication aids, something familiar and unthreatening that carries an unmistakable message about what is really important to us. In the case of the literature we are considering, really important to everybody.

Written texts exist in themselves; they are there to be used. They will not go away as soon as the performance is over. They can be glanced over or studied in depth – read or learned. You can even read them several times over, if you have time. You can read them by yourself or with other people. If you do this aloud, individuals can take separate roles, which can be read straight through or swapped over in mid-stream. You can, of course, identify with the characters, as you do in all drama. This usually happens with the character you yourself are reading at the time, but people frequently become imaginatively involved with other characters in the play. In fact, reading plays in this way creates its own kind of atmosphere. People are involved with the whole activity of sharing a text together. It is as if the play itself takes over; we are involved in the world created by the author and preserved on the page ready to be brought vibrantly to life in the imagination of the people reading it.

The gap between making a scene up and learning lines beforehand is actually less dramatic, less frightening, than people usually assume it to be. The same thing turns out to be true with regard to the difference between reading plays and actually performing them. As everyone knows who has ever taken part in, or been a member of the audience at, a public play reading, such an event 'comes across' as a genuine performance in its own right, as the readers take on the roles as if the things imagined by the author were actually happening – *and they were the people they were happening to* – and the quality of their involvement in what they are imagining communicates itself to the audience so that, as in a theatre, everybody's imagination takes wing. Acting in a play, extemporising a scene or reading a text are all basically drama; all depend on cancelling out the division between performers and spectators or listeners by creating a situation in which all such differences are removed, and what would otherwise be barriers between us turn out to be grist to the mill of our dramatic imaginations.

From this point of view, then, the written text turns out to be nearer to the actual performance than we may have assumed it to be, as our imagination carries out the job it does so well, that of leaping the gap between different spheres of reality and allowing us to form relationships which at first sight appear unlikely or even impossible. Up to now we have been concentrating our attention on improvised drama and drama-therapeutic approaches that do not involve the actual written texts of plays. It turns out, however, that there is not all that much to choose between these two experiences: improvised drama can be spontaneous and immediate, but so can doing dramatherapy from a text, if you are willing to let yourself go along with what you are reading and use your imagination.

In fact, there are some situations in which using the text of a play may be the better approach. One which immediately comes to mind is where the members of the group are not able to move around as freely as they would like to. They may be physically immobilised or wheelchair-bound or confined to their beds. This does not mean that improvising is impossible from such a position (although it does seem easier when you can show what you are imagining in the way that your bodies are positioned with regard to each other and don't have to rely on words and gestures alone); but the presence of the written text acts as a focus point for the imagination, a kind of meeting place which we use to distract all our attention from our immediate situation. Here again, it is imagination which makes it work; and when you are 'playing from the text', the book is literally as well as metaphorically something to hold on to. There are other reasons, too, for wanting to hold on to the book. People can be shy and not want to move around; at least not at first, until they know one another better and can relax more. Some people, too, regard drama as essentially an intellectual sphere of activity, and do not feel that they are taking it seriously unless they can have a written text and preferably one by an author they have heard of. This is usually something instilled into them at school and can consequently be difficult to shift. If this is the view of the group as a whole it might be advisable to go with the flow and start off with a written text, whatever may happen afterwards!

These are rather negative reasons for using text in dramatherapy, and they could be regarded as trying to make the best of a bad job. There are more positive indications for a text-centred approach. The most important of these is the opportunity provided to look at the play as a whole, and to take in what the author has to say. Unless it is possible to arrange for all the members of a dramatherapy group to visit a theatre together, working from the text is the only way in which the impact of a complete play as written by the author can be experienced. Even though it may not always be immediately obvious to everybody present in the theatre, plays are always intended to be *about* something. Once this underlying theme has been grasped, certain parts of the play leap to people's attention as crucially important for the drama as a whole, and these can be explored dramatherapeutically as a springboard for dramatic work of various kinds within the session itself. Reading the play, immersing yourself in the world it conjures up, has the effect of raising issues that are of personal concern not only to the author and the characters she or he has created, but also to you, the reader. This does not mean they are matters you are always concerned with and find yourself thinking about. They may actually be things that you do not really want to think about at all and usually manage to avoid considering in any great depth. Once the matter has been brought up in this way, however, so that all of a sudden you find yourself personally involved in what is happening to these people, then 'the play's the thing' for you; the whole play, not simply an episode from it, although it was this particular episode or event or situation within it that first brought it to life for you.

We recognise ourselves in the play as a whole – the story, the setting, the people involved. Thinking about it in retrospect, we find ourselves running over the whole story, playing all the roles in our imagination. From a psychotherapeutic point of view this can be a healing experience, as we recognise different sides of our own personality in the different characters of the drama. This is not as straightforward as it sounds. As we said, there are things about ourselves we might prefer to forget; psychological reactions that we have trained ourselves not to recognise as integral parts of our unconscious life, having managed to detach them from our consciousness at an early stage of our psychological development. Having time to study the play as a whole may bring us face to face with these unwelcome aspects of ourselves.

The dramatherapy approach, then, may concentrate on bringing to life particular parts of the whole, so that the whole comes alive in a new way. The parts of the play that are chosen by the group as a whole, or by individual members of it, are ones in which the central dramatic theme, the main thrust, of the play stands out more clearly. They are the things which seem to sum up what it is all about. Because a principal aim of drama-therapy is the uncovering of hidden conflicts, the plays chosen for this kind of work are usually ones whose main theme concerns areas of life which give rise to psychological pain and social conflict. It does not have to go out of its way to do this. Many of the greatest plays in dramatic literature are about these things; indeed it is hard to say how a play could be considered great unless it had something to say regarding the things that are really important about life, and the really important things which always carry with them the risk of involving us in difficult situations. There are several ways that drama can deal with this basic fact, as, for example, comedy, tragedy, farce, satire, romance or straightforward documentary. A play does not have to 'carry its heart on its sleeve', announcing its theme immediately in the first few scenes, and its final effect may be quite different from what we were expecting it to be – sadder, happier, more thoughtful, more personal – but we will not discover this until we have finished reading it, any more than we can say precisely how we shall be feeling when we leave the theatre, although we thought we knew very well what to expect before the play started! Plays aim at being complete statements, even when they leave us wondering what will happen next to the people whose lives we have been observing. Taken in themselves they are genuine happenings, with a beginning, a middle and an end, even though they may be about people nothing seems to be happening to. (A good example would be Samuel Beckett's *Waiting for Godot*, but some of Chekhov's plays also fit this category.)

A list of well-known plays chosen at random reminds us that each of them is built round or constructed upon a specific life-theme. Each play has other themes, of course. Imaginative literature uses acted or written stories to present human experience in a way that is able to take account of all its richness, and not simply to transmit a single message or embody only one viewpoint. Each play has many voices and this is what makes it lifelike. Because plays show human society as the setting for all kinds of conflicting attitudes and interests, they are more like debates than lectures or sermons. But this is the unique power of drama. Out of the many points of view clamouring for attention, one voice wins the day, so that we can say with some conviction that this is, for us at least, what this play is 'about'.

Here are some examples. Each of the following plays could be said to be mainly about the quality, attitude or value stated. This is an entirely personal view, of course. Playwrights are not in the habit of explaining their work in such an obvious way. The purpose of making such a list is to demonstrate how it is possible to form a judgement with regard to what a particular play is about. Judgements will always differ. Part of the process of working on written texts from a dramatherapy point of view is the effort to come to a decision about what the main message of a play may be. All kinds of different conclusions offer themselves to be explored. Here are some chosen more or less at random:

| | | |
|---|---|---|
| *Oedipus Rex* | Sophocles | Responsibility/identity |
| *Everyman* | Traditional morality play | The human condition |
| *Dr Faustus* | Marlowe | Power through knowledge |
| *Macbeth* | Shakespeare | Ambition/nemesis |
| *Hamlet* | Shakespeare | The courage to be |
| *King Lear* | Shakespeare | Learning to love |
| *Othello* | Shakespeare | Insecurity/treachery |
| *Romeo and Juliet* and *Antony and Cleopatra* | Shakespeare | The freedom to love/ the power of passion |
| *Twelfth Night* | Shakespeare | The quest for love |
| *The Tempest* | Shakespeare | Growth and change |
| *Tartuffe* | Molière | Deceit and manipulation |
| *The School for Scandal* | Sheridan | Social pretence versus genuine human feelings |
| *Hedda Gabler* | Ibsen | Hidden guilt |
| *The Cherry Orchard* | Chekhov | Looking backwards, clinging to the past |
| *The Good Woman of Sechzuan* | Brecht | Social exploitation |
| *Waiting for Godot* | Beckett | The search for meaning |

These are all plays from the standard theatrical repertoire. What we are saying does not apply only to well-known plays. Life-themes can be drawn from all kinds of drama. Some kinds of plays are particularly useful as vehicles for presenting the individual histories of members of the group, or the corporate life story of the group as a whole. Written texts, actual plays, are experienced as being more safe than extemporised ones, perhaps because the play's author takes responsibility for the things that happen in it. A good example of this is the work done by dramatherapy groups on *The Revenger's Tragedy* (1607) – a Jacobean play which is removed from current experience through time, genre, form and class and so provides the cast with unparalleled opportunities for 'coming clean' with regard to unacknowledged aspects of their own personal dramas (Andersen-Warren 1991). Horror plays, adventure plays full of amazing events and reversals of fortune, whose far-fetched theatrical nature makes them appear at first sight to be more of an excuse for having fun at one another's – and the audience's – expense rather than a serious investigation into 'real' states of mind, provide a container for feelings, attitudes, relationships and situations which might otherwise prove too threatening for the group to approach head-on.

To use a written text in this way is to approach it in a more focused, more specifically therapeutic manner than simply using it as a springboard for presenting one's own personal dramas, although this in itself can be a creative thing to do. Looked at as a whole, a play is a powerful way of typifying a specific kind of human interpersonal experience. The personages involved in its story, however, behave as individuals as well as human cogs in the machinery of the plot. They provide us with examples of human behaviour which we can relate to our own experience. We can identify with this, remain aloof from it, or reject it out of hand. Or, as often happens, we can be in two minds about it, openly repudiating it while secretly recognising our own collusive involvement in whatever is going on, even though we may not approve of it at all, of course. In dramatherapy which uses the written text of a play, the characters are there for us to take our time thinking about and pondering over. The presence of the text itself gives us the opportunity to take to heart the people in it – not in the same immediate way that we do in the theatre, but more reflectively, more thoughtfully.

To sum up, then, text-based dramatherapy gives us time to think about the women and men we are becoming imaginatively involved with – and consequently to think about *ourselves*. Marina Jenkyns (1996) describes how using text allows us to concentrate on the unacknowledged parts of ourselves as these are personified by the characters in the play. As I read the written text, I am able to become more and more aware of these emotions and action pathways which chime with aspects of my own psychological life. This is in itself a healing experience. As Jenkyns says, 'A play can provide healing precisely because it provides a place to which people can bring the unconscious text of their own lives, and by meeting the form and structure of the play, find new ways to shape their experience' (Jenkyns 1996, p.72). The function of 'shaping experience' is one of *psychological containment*. This happens when we are actually performing plays where 'what we have is the actor projecting part of himself, by means of a character, into the part of himself which can act that character, so that it can be both contained and acted out, held and expressed' (Jenkyns 1996, pp.48, 49). It is also, however, an important function of reading plays too:

> It is not uncommon to work with a text onto which a group can project its own unwanted feelings such as hate and fear, loss and vulnerability – they will say the text is awful, horrible, depressing, the parts are the last things they want to play – yet through the process of working on it, the group members both grow closer together and allow the play to work for them as it allows them safely to acknowledge these things of darkness. (Jenkyns 1996, p.45)

From an object-relations point of view, dramatherapy may be seen as a way of reincorporating those parts of the self which have become 'split off' (to use Melanie Klein's (1988) term) as a defensive measure during early childhood. Although this process of reconstruction is considered to be largely unconscious, it needs to be consciously recognised and systematically worked on – which is why having the text available for study is an obvious advantage.

In dramatherapy, the crucial stage of working with a text is the point when readers become actors. Actual performance of the plays makes up the central stage of a dramatherapeutic process, and the theatrical face of dramatherapy which we have been looking at in previous chapters, the healing power of dramatic distance, comes into its own using material specially prepared for it – parts that have been worked on by the actors, a play that has been carefully constructed to have maximum dramatic force, now presented as a real piece of theatre: '...the play is the raw material and the finished product' (Andersen-Warren 1996, p.134). This does not only apply to the texts of plays which have already been written and performed elsewhere, of course. Andersen-Warren (1996) describes a group creating their own version of a well-known play and performing it before an audience drawn from the public. The process falls into three parts, but the creative action is there from the beginning, as the play makes use of an already existing dramatic situation and develops it by working on it during rehearsal, then presents it as a living experience in performance and finally moves out of the play 'frame' altogether, as performers and audience take time to share their ideas and feelings about what it has been like to look at life through the medium of theatre. This, too, is 'working from the text' – the text in this case is one evolved from the living experience of those taking part (Andersen-Warren 1996; Grainger 1999b).

## A descriptive study of a dramatherapy group centred on a group's experience of seeing *The Revenger's Tragedy*

*Tourneur's* The Revenger's Tragedy *(Gibbon 1967) may not seem to be one of the most obvious choices for the beginning of dramatherapeutic work, dealing as it does with the darker and more savage aspects of human nature. However, the shadows and darkness of the play provided a catalyst, a dark gestation from which new perceptions can emerge.*

The setting for the group work was within a small psychiatric unit in a general hospital in the North of England.

This was to be the background for the forging of links between theatre and therapy. Two things in particular made the task possible. First, it had been supported by managers who had allowed financial support for theatre visits. The participants were, therefore, familiar with the conventions of theatre. Second, all of the group members had prior experience in dramatherapy groups with the author (Madeline Anderson-Warren). The hospital had involvement with community theatre groups, local theatres and artists.

Several clients had expressed an interest in the Royal Shakespeare Company as they had heard about it from a variety of media sources. Many of them had seen and enjoyed performances of Shakespeare's plays and were interested in seeing some of the less frequently performed plays by his contemporaries. Guided by these criteria, a trip to the Swan Theatre was organised to see *The Revenger's Tragedy* (Gibbon 1967).

At the time of the visit the 12 group members, aged between 23 and 62, were attending the psychiatric day hospital, industrial units or community mental health care centres. A diagnosis of psychotic disorder had been made. None were in an acute, florid stage but all had some evidence of psycho-motor retardation and rigidity, concrete thinking, and thought disorder. Grainger (1990) describes the perceptional disorders as being 'like spectators at a football match who can only see a very limited section of the field and keep being expected to join in the game. Their inability to step outside themselves and observe the match from someone else's viewpoint means they never know which angle the ball is coming from next' (Grainger 1990, p.53).

Dramatherapy work had already helped to extend the clients' aware-ness of body boundaries; that is, the relationships between their own body parts and those between self and other. It was hoped that the new programme for the group would further extend their perceptions of reality by working with dramatic reality.

Before the theatre visit we spent one session talking about the play, becoming familiar with its language and characters. The text abounds with references to the brevity of life – a joke with death as the punch line – and there are recurrent images of the macabre grinning skull behind the countenance of soft flesh. The semi-allegorical characters mock, jest and joke about death, decay, decadence, disease and violence.

The style of the writing alternates between comic, quick-fire, alliter-ative lines like Spurio's reaction to hearing of his father's death, 'Old dad dead?' (Gibbon 1967, v.i.109), and slow meditative soliloquies during which Vindice, the protagonist, broods on thoughts of evil and injustice. So far as the plot goes, the play is a farce, a satirical riot of vitality and juxtaposition. The characters rumble and romp through their plots and counterplots of revenge, retribution, power and corruption. These are plays which have the lurid fascination of half-remembered nightmares. At the same time, one is trying to recall the dream while also trying to forget and push away the frightening images.

The group's enjoyment of the play was tremendous. The production encompassed the whole theatre, with the actors moving freely around the stalls and balconies. The costumes were elaborate and, coupled with the frenetic action, made the performance visually exciting. Along with the clarity and tone of the actors' speech, these visual stimuli provoked a willing suspension of disbelief in the group. They became engrossed in the action, often pointing to people to warn them about their impending doom. Rather than recoiling from the spectacle they responded as if they were at a pantomime – a reaction in keeping with the atmosphere generated by the performance.

Whether they fully understood the complicated plots did not matter. They had been moved by a series of strong images and were conscious of having a vivid experience of chaos, safely contained within a dramatic structure played out on a stage.

This became evident on the journey home. In the security of the warm coach they talked with fervour of the deeds they had witnessed. This was something new to them – evidence of their own fears and inner chaos, presented theatrically in a different and external form. The fact that they had seen it together put a seal on the experience.

The first group was held four days after the visit and was to continue over ten weeks as a closed group.

The dramatherapist recorded that

> The group was fascinated and intrigued by the terrors and violence of the play. They described their reactions and responses in terms of the 'horrid laughter' that Nicholas Brook describes in his book of the same name (1979). They are also slightly puzzled by their mirth at the horrendous acts. They cite the sight of Vindice and Hippolito breaking the dead duke's fingers to fit round a goblet in particular. I need to enable them to explore the chaos and darker aspects without them becoming engulfed in the darkness with no way out.

She decided to start with the visual aspects of the play and not to work directly from the text, as several members were not literate.

### Session 1

As the five females and seven males gather for the group they are still talking about the play and are exchanging memories in a random way. After re-setting the ground rules we complete some warm-up work to free the body and to focus energies.

We begin by retracing our steps from the Swan Theatre foyer to the point of finding our seats. Doing this reunites us as a group with a common focus, and also involves us in a small ritual. This is necessarily slow, before entering into the frenzy of the play. The aim is to establish a 'place of safety' for the group, so that they have a place where they can become watchers or observers of their own action – a place where they become distanced while still being involved in the drama. From our position as 'audience' we recall the play and decided upon the stage area in the room.

From here we divide into three groups of four to produce sculpted images of the play. One group wants to explore the setting, so we divide the play into three sections: one group to take the first third, the second the second third, and the other the final section.

- *The first group* chooses the first scene of the play and shows Vindice kneeling with the skull in his hand. Two courtiers stand and mock him.

- *The second group* shows the jailer holding the severed head while the two brothers of the deceased stand jesting and laughing.

- *The third group* shows the Duchess about to be banished. The character in charge of this stands holding her wig, while a third person, from the court, points at the bald woman and enjoys her indignity.

- *The final group* reproduces the array of candles that had burned throughout the performance at the Swan.

We then move to the adding of words to the tableaux. The majority of people make clear statements about something being taken from them:

Duchess:   My wig is being snatched – I am exposed for an old, ugly woman. How will I survive my banishment?

Jailer:    I am stuck with holding someone else's head – I am frightened of losing mine.

Courtier (*about Vindice*): I see he is holding a head – maybe he will take mine.

The hopeful and positive statements were from the last group:

Candle:    I see terrible things but I continue to burn.

The statements offered by the first three groups contain possible connect-ions with colloquialisms relating to madness – 'off his/her rocker/head'; 'losing my head/mind' – and also with other vulnerabilities and issues. They might be interpreted as dramatic metaphors dealing with the closure of the local large psychiatric hospital, or clients' experiences of their own discharges from institutions.

We close by all joining the candle group and forming a 'macro-sculpt'. Each person describes what they see on the 'stage' and says what help they can offer from their static position. Hope, faith and light are the most popular choices. We reflect on the drama from our places in the audience and then remove ourselves further by going to an area outside both 'audience' and 'stage' positions to finish the session.

*THERAPIST'S THOUGHTS AND REFLECTIONS*

*I feel that the 'candles' sculpt can provide us with the image of shadow oppositions and work as a useful focus for the start of the next session. Its stillness provides a calmness. Symbolically, candles are linked with rituals connected with birth, death, celebration and mourning. I am reminded of the lines from* Waiting for Godot, *'they give birth astride of a grave; the light gleams an instant, then its night once more' (Beckett 1986, p.83). I formulate the idea of working with the candle gleam as a central concept, looking backwards and forwards, creating the light and the shade.*

*Playtext linking with playtext, one playwright adding to another, often provides inspiration for dramatherapeutic work. Jennings (1990) explains this process thus: 'Whereas psychotherapists will often recall particular theorists or case histories, dramatherapists recall themes from dramatic works of art – plays, performances, myths, images, metaphors, symbols' (1990, p.57). So, the next session focused on 'gleam'.*

### Session 2

The group arrives, still reminiscing about the play. After the warm-up work, which is an extension of the space–place explorations we started last week, the candle tableau is reformed.

A theme emerges: the candles can 'see' in two directions. Looking one way they can see the court, the chaos, the harsh glitter and the decay. I ask for words and the word 'worm' becomes important, a word often spoken in the play. The group offer 'silkworm'; 'the worms that eat you up when you are dead'; 'worming your way up'; 'tape-worm'; 'sitting in the garden eating worms'.

I ask the group to remain with the worm imagery but to turn and look in the other direction; what can they see outside the court? If the stage set can be extended what would the other place be? What are the other functions of worms? Does the light of the candles become stronger? They offer the suggestion that there is a country place where the worms turn the soil to keep the soil fertile and enable the crops to grow.

To finish this session we discuss how it feels to be still and see both sides of the situation. We work within the metaphor of 'throwing light on the matter'.

THERAPIST'S THOUGHTS AND REFLECTIONS

*My perceptions are that the group members are starting to extend their fields of vision. In relation to Grainger's analogy of the football field, to bring both goals into vision (Grainger 1990).*

### Sessions 3 and 4

We create the set for our drama using cardboard boxes, coloured paper, foil, string, chicken wire, different textures of material and paint. Slowly, and with great concentration, the room is transformed and the imagined forms become actual. The area designated as the stage becomes the court. Chairs are covered with foil and decorated with velvet and braids. Wooden poles are decorated to form abstract gaudy structures and are joined using string. The predominant colours are red, gold and black. At the back of the court a cardboard structure is built and candles made from crêpe paper are glued on to separate the court from the country. The country set is green, yellow and blue with crêpe paper flowers and a few poles painted in stripes of blue and white. Brightly coloured banners are hung from the poles, creating an atmosphere of celebration.

The group members co-operate and debate while working, and they form all the design ideas. I offer advice and help with technical matters, bearing in mind that we will need to take the set apart after each session and quickly reassemble it as the room is used for other groups. On completion, we take our 'audience' places and discuss the set. Again, the group focuses on the central candles and discusses their function as sources of light and illumination.

### Session 5

We are already at our halfway point. The court, candles, worms and set are established as important and powerful dramatic metaphors within which group members can experiment with different ways of being and perceiving the self, others and the environment.

We begin by discussing the types of people who might live in the country. We start from the worms. This provides ideas about country dwellers being earthy people who toil and tend the land. Individuals start to form their own characters whom we name. We have farmers, a miller, peasants, labourers and brewers. We explore how the characters move, how their clothes affect the movement, how they show their emotions, what sounds they make and what their needs are. The time and place is decided: it is the evening of the Harvest Festival. We create the celebration using the banners and flowers.

When the characters rest I introduce the idea that they have heard about some events at the Duke's court and gossip about them. I remind the group of some of the events at the start of the play: the younger son's trial for raping the good Antonio's wife; her resulting suicide; the power struggles and plots.

THERAPIST'S THOUGHTS AND REFLECTIONS
*This created both distance and a way in – a solid ordinary viewpoint on the chaos and disruption. With this particular client group the aim was to build into the drama a choice of safety nets.*

*Session 6*

We move to creating the court characters. We negotiate parts. Spurio, the character perhaps most open to and aware of his own evil, is the most popular choice. The group insists that we only have one person per character, and reject the suggestion that we can have a 'multiple Spurio' with different people playing different aspects of him – 'greed', 'power', 'lust'.

Parts are finally negotiated. Some people elect to play courtiers and nobles. We discard the sub-plot with Vindice's mother and sisters because they are described as 'living outside the court' and people cannot remember them well. Someone brings up the problems of language and how difficult it will be to reproduce the feel of the text without poetry, or 'old words' as he expresses it. We decide to work with mime, as the patients are quite experienced at using the body as the major vehicle of expression. After some character formation work, we move slowly through the play.

As we progress, the representation becomes more frantic, tense and grotesque, echoing, while not actually reproducing, the moves of the witnessed performance. What is important is that the theatre experience has provided a new language and style in which people can express themselves, an addition to their own imaginations. Through the dramatic distance they are able to explore the shadows and darker aspects of the experience.

At the end of the session I de-role the group, moving them back to everyday reality via the country scene and encouraging them to reflect on the drama we have performed.

### Session 7

We decide which section of the play we want to explore further. The group chooses the final scene, which includes most of the cast. Characters such as the Duke and Duchess, who are dead or banished, decide to take up my suggestion that they can be at the side of the stage, in character, as witnesses. The group plays the scene in slow motion to extend and exaggerate movement and also to prevent injury in the presentation of the various stabbings that take place. (The device also serves to preserve detail without destroying spontaneity.) Once this is completed I ask the group to divide into three subgroups to discuss their ideal endings to the play.

At the end of Tourneur's play [Gibbon 1967] the good nobleman Antonio emerges as the new Duke. Most of the other characters have been killed, and he sends Vindice and his brother to be executed for all the murders they have committed. The group agrees that Antonio should not rule as the new Duke and that he, too, should be killed. They argue that he, too, will turn out to be wicked. Indeed, he displays his unsuitability for just rule in that his first action as Duke is to send people to their deaths.

THERAPIST'S THOUGHTS AND REFLECTIONS

*The group members are stuck, having no ideas of how to move forward. They don't want the play to end with the stage littered with corpses, without any living beings, nor do they want any of their characters to survive. In their stuckness they are silent. Because of this, I suggested that they move into the 'audience' place and say the names of things that are on the stage. They become slowly reanimated, listing tables, chairs, candles, dishes and goblets from the banquet, fruit, masks from a masque and so on. I ask them to re-engage with the country characters and to reflect on the court devastation. They conclude that the answers will be found in the masks. Thus, by means of the dramatic process, they contact their own inner knowing and wisdom.*

### Session 8

We make masks from card and scraps of material. These are flat masks attached to bamboo poles, designed to be held at distance from the face. (As we have only a further two sessions I do not feel it is appropriate to introduce full facial masks. These would take us into different dimensions of dramatic reality, and would have taken more time to work with.)

This form of mask also gives us the opportunity to make the mask double-sided. One side is the mask of the treacherous character, dancing in a masque with the sinister purpose of murder. The other is the progression after the final scene of the play. Again we are dealing with the duality of light and dark. When the masks are completed we move with the 'court' side on the outside. Although some people are performing the dance with discordant, chaotic and sinister movement, their own view is of the brighter, inner aspect.

We return, once again, to our 'audience' positions and talk about the dance. Many references are made to the 'dance of death' and the way the sight of the other masks dancing was 'a bit scary', and how reassuring it was to be able to put the mask to the side sometimes, or to have the view of one's own inner mask.

### Session 9

We again focus on the dance of chaos and destruction before moving into the 'candle area' to experience stillness and calm. The masks are reversed to show movement into the country area, where a circle dance of joy celebrates the changing seasons.

During the feedback session the group discusses how important it is to have both sides of the mask. They feel that they represent union of the two sides. The fact that they were holding the masks allowed them to feel in control. I remind them of some of the statements they made in the first session, about 'losing heads', and they compare the feelings contained in the sculpts with the control they now feel. They also focus on the importance of the candles as a mid-point. We keep the discussion within the dramatic metaphor as new insights are continually emerging because of dramatic distance.

*Session 10*

The group says goodbye to the masks and the candles. They decide what messages, feelings and thoughts they will take with them and what they will, symbolically, leave behind. We have a final reflection on past sessions and then slowly dismantle the set for the last time. The group leaves as individuals who have shared an important journey with others.

As I reflect on the group I am aware, as I was at the time, of all the rich possibilities for exploring the multitude of pathways that the group members offered. The play was always our focus. Although the time spent on the actual representation of the text was not lengthy in relation to time spent on other areas, the images and concepts of the Stratford performance were the inspiration for all our images. The total impact of the production informed the thinking and imagination of the group, the movement, the set, the props, the lighting and the dance. The most difficult area for the group was the text. It would have been possible to work directly with the text, to analyse some speeches and isolate some key points in the play, but I decided, rightly or wrongly, to concentrate on the movement within the dramatic structure. I would argue that this further increased the power of the drama.

This world of the drama had permitted a sharing of different forms of reality, an exploration of the group's own terrors via a setting far removed in time, class and place. Sometimes group members explicitly made their own links, but mostly the real fiction of dramatic reality rendered the links implicit and thus safer to explore.

## Working with text

*A group of ten people with abnormal grief reactions, who were experiencing 'stuckness and a sense of denial' – unable to express their terrible sense of loss.*

*The therapist suggested lines from Shakespeare's* Twelfth Night *(Act II, scene iv):*

> *...she pin'd in thought*
> *And with a green and yellow melancholy*
> *She sat like Patience on a monument,*
> *Smiling at grief.*

*Although these lines are actually about unrequited love, they seemed to be applicable to the group state.*

*Introduction*

When the lines were read to the group members they were silent for a while. When one person asked to hear them again, others nodded. As they heard the words for the second time everyone was attentive. Several people said how surprised they were that their feelings were expressed so well by a person who lived so long ago.

*Structure*

The structures implemented over the six two-hour sessions were:

1   Painting the 'green and yellow melancholy'. These pictures were put together and viewed by the group participants. Looking at them from various angles, they came to the conclusion that they looked like a swamp. This swamp image became a symbol of the feelings of stuckness the group were experiencing. They were able to engage in expressions of feelings about sinking and feeling unsafe.

2   The image of 'Patience on a monument, smiling at grief' became a powerful structure for their own entanglement and inability to 'move away' from the deceased person.

> First, people drew a picture of Patience, smiling at her grief. People felt that they were both part of the monument and onlookers.

> Next, the group made dramatic sculpts or images of each monument, each person portraying the figure of Patience in his or her own monument.

> Each person then portrayed Patience away from the monument, saying why she was 'smiling at grief'.

*This enabled a moving forward from the process of denial. The struggle to carry on smiling had resulted in holding on to emotion and keeping it private. Many people feared they would be perceived as weak, vulnerable or a 'burden' if they actually expressed the way they felt.*

3   The monument images were drawn, this time with a different figure in place of Patience. People were able to create a monument for the deceased person and allow 'goodbyes' to be expressed.

# CHAPTER 9

# Assessment and Evaluation

## How Can We Tell if Dramatherapy
## Is or Has Been Effective?

The aim of this short chapter is to say something about the way we make judgements about the success or failure of the dramatherapy we have been doing – in other words, the ways we evaluate it. The subject is important at several different levels. It is obviously very relevant if the intention is to carry out formal research into the way that dramatherapy works – or to establish on a more definite basis the fact that it *does* work. There is obviously no justification in wasting time and money and building up people's hopes of a successful outcome if it can be demonstrated that the dramatherapy approach has no positive effects or that it actually makes things worse! Nowadays tremendous stress is laid on the scientific testing of therapeutic approaches, partly because of a growing awareness of the rights of patients – who have such faith in the skill and wisdom of the medical authorities they turn to for help – and partly because of the extremely widespread and well-established opinion that nothing has any valid public reality unless it can be explained in a scientific way using scientific language. Some attempts have been made to bring dramatherapy, along with the other 'arts therapies', safely into the world of science. We shall be mentioning these later on.

First things first, however. You, as a practitioner, have to have ways of deciding whether things are going well or badly both during and after an individual session and over a whole course of dramatherapy. You need more than a vague feeling of satisfaction or discouragement when the question of success or failure is raised – which, of course, it is bound to be, both privately and in public. First of all, however, you have to know what, for you, 'going well' means. You must yourself have arrived at some kind of

definition of therapeutic success. In terms of the task-orientated dramatherapy we were looking at in Chapter 2, success and failure have already
been made quite specific in terms of the function of a particular agency
with which you are associated – members of an assertiveness group, for
instance, either become more able to assert themselves as a result of the
dramatherapy they have been taking part in, or they do not. This is
something that can actually be measured by psychometric tests.

This kind of clarity is not always achievable, however. The overall aim
of dramatherapy could be described as the improvement of people's ability
to make emotional and cognitive sense of themselves and their
surroundings. This is a very vague way of talking about the things which
constitute human psychological well-being; in order to be able to feel that
dramatherapy is actually having some kind of identifiable beneficial effect,
we have to operationalise it in terms of actual changes taking place in
people's behaviour and experience. Dramatherapy has to be meaningful
for everyone involved. If it is not for the practitioner, it certainly will not
be for the patients or clients.

In other words, we must know what we are looking for – what actual
healing consists of in any particular case. Only when you have settled this
to your own (and others') satisfaction can you be in a position to take the
necessary steps towards drawing conclusions as to whether it has come
about or not. Knowing that the therapy has worked is not the same as
knowing *how* it works. This will certainly need some kind of special
investigation. One thing is certain, however. You will not recognise the
processes involved unless you have a real sense of the end to be achieved.
You may not be able to express this sense in so many words, and our
experience of dramatherapy leads us to believe that the ability to form
conclusions of this kind 'before the event', so that we know exactly what it
is we are looking for, is not always necessary. 'I don't know what we're
trying to do,' said a member of a dramatherapy group to the partner with
whom he was struggling to construct a dramatic scenario. 'Never mind,'
his friend said, 'You won't know what it is until you do it.' The
dramatherapist immediately jotted this down: it seemed such a good
description of her own experience.

## Coding the process

Therapists working with groups – and this includes dramatherapists, of course – are often conscious of a need to capture the group drama as it is being played out rather than having to depend on words, looks and phrases which they have managed to remember, plus an overall sense of 'the way things went', which is all that can often be salvaged once the session is over. Nowadays it is quite common for sessions to be recorded on videotape and this is assumed to result in the most accurate version of events that may reasonably be hoped for. In one way, however, the very accuracy of video recordings may be a distraction from what actually went on in the group. In group experience things are not always exactly as they appear; or rather, there is a lot that can be visually and aurally recorded, and also a good deal that cannot. Therapists who depend entirely on tapes can be just as conscious that more happened in a particular session than met the eye of the video camera.

What cannot be accurately recorded by mechanisms is the inner life of a group, what Murray Cox has called 'the empathetic quality of shared humanity' (1978, p.37). This is why you may find it more satisfactory to work out your own way of gauging how successful a dramatherapy session has been. The history of group therapy provides many examples of attempts to codify the dynamic interactions that take place both among the group members themselves and between individuals or subgroups and the therapist or therapists, either during the course of a session or over a course of sessions. Foulkes and Anthony were among the first to attempt to do this (1957, pp.101–105). Later on, Murray Cox (1978) devised a way of recording dynamic aspects of therapeutic group interaction which allowed him to pinpoint exactly what kinds of interpersonal events he, as a psychodynamic therapist, considered to be crucial for therapy. This involved the use of what he called VDS (Visual Display Systems), which provide a kind of shorthand way of noting down particular aspects of therapeutic sessions while not getting distracted by things that the therapist considers to be less important (Cox 1978). Here again, it is the therapist's judgement that matters. Only you can decide what sort of thing you are looking for, but you may find you need the framework provided by your system of notation, perhaps in the form of a visual plan in which you can record fluctuations of relationship and changes of intention and emotional tone within the group in the shape of some kind of diagram you yourself have thought up for the purpose. The most important thing, however, is to know what it is you are looking for, what kind of change you yourself consider to be significant, and to have a convenient way of recording the occurrence. For some people, there remains no substitute for the effort to write up the session as it came across to them. In fact, however, this can be the most accurate way of keeping in touch with the quality of emotional and relational changes which happened within the group. The distancing required in order to write the session up allows some of the feelings to become more accessible. As we saw, this kind of distance lets us feel the emotional reality of things which we are unconsciously defended against.

## Supervision

One way of evaluating your work is to ask someone else whose opinion you respect to share your experience with you. People who work professionally as dramatherapists are supervised by other professionals, either fellow arts therapists or others involved in psychological healing of one kind or another. 'Supervision,' say Shohet and Hawkins, 'offers a framework where professional experience can be survived, reflected upon and learnt from' (1989, p.3). Some dramatherapists prefer to be supervised by their fellows; but not everybody requires the person supervising them to be as familiar with dramatherapeutic techniques as they are themselves. This is because of the way supervision works. Shohet and Hawkins (1989) have demonstrated that it has less to do with intellectual criticism than with the exploration of client–therapist relationships. What comes to the surface in a supervision session is the quality of interpersonal happenings within the therapy session which is being described by the therapist. In a very real sense, therapy sessions are relived in supervision sessions, although in a very different way, one which can permit greater clarity of understanding on the part of the therapist who is now able to relive her or his feelings within an environment which is detached from the actual therapy. Because these emotions are actually relived and not simply talked about, their reality is understood and appreciated by the supervisor, enabling him or her to gain a vivid personal understanding of what the actual therapy session was like. At the same time, however, the supervisor is more detached from the original events than the supervisee. Searles

(1965) describes a process whereby the 'therapeutic distance' between client and therapist is reinforced by that between therapist and supervisor, giving rise to a sharing of emotional insights that preserve the truth of the original event without defensive distortions. Thus the supervisor is able to encourage the supervisees to sit back and take real stock of their feelings so that they can return to the therapy group with an increased sense of their own ability to contain the emotions which will be focused on them there, emotions which can be realised and used only therapeutically, in terms of their own ability to respond to them.

Dramatherapists need supervision for the same reason as other psychotherapists – because they are exposed to situations of extreme psychological distress. Although supervisors may, and often do, give practical advice, their evaluations tend to be psychological; in other words, they are empathetic explorations of the therapist's experience within the group rather than technical judgements as to whether a particular approach can be considered successful or not, or what it is that actually constitutes success in dramatherapy. This kind of evaluation remains largely the responsibility of individual practitioners. Generally speaking, if you are a dramatherapist – or in fact any other kind of psychotherapist – you have to find your own way to judge the success or failure of the work you are doing. Nobody can really do this for you, because in the long run it depends entirely on your own personal stance, the way that you, as a person, make sense of life. Before you can begin to be a professional therapist you must be reasonably clear in your mind on two very important questions which govern the practice of all kinds of therapeutic activity. The first of these concerns the nature of personal healing. What, in your view, constitutes this? The second question is closely associated with the first: what, then, are you willing to take as evidence of its presence? Other people's judgements on these matters are of very great importance. Indeed, they always have to be taken into account in whatever you decide to do in order to evaluate your own work, as we shall be discussing in the next section; but unless *you yourself know* what it is you are looking for and *how you will be able to tell that you have found it* you will never really be able to evaluate any kind of therapy you become involved in. Other people's judgements are always very important, but never so important as your own sense of what actually constitutes evidence about the truth.

## Formal evaluation

This kind of ongoing awareness of purpose and progress might be called 'informal evaluation'. Sometimes it is conscious, often it is the unexpressed basis of the assumptions we make about therapy. You are recommended, however, to make it less informal by finding your own way of mapping your therapeutic journey and recording your progress in it, so that your practice may be more 'evidence-based'.

Actual research, however, is by definition a lot more formal and systematic than this. *The Concise Oxford Dictionary* defines it as 'Formulated knowledge; the pursuit of knowledge or the principles regulating such pursuit; organised body of knowledge' and *Chambers Dictionary* as 'Knowledge ascertained by observation and experiment, critically tested and brought under general principles'. In practice, research means testing observations against what you believe to be reality and making some attempt to communicate your findings to other people. This almost certainly involves a process of drawing conclusions about the things you are examining and then going through a process of successively discarding them in favour of new ones until you are satisfied that you have identified the nature of the phenomena under scrutiny. As Gordon Langley puts it, 'Knowledge is refined through a sense of approximations each with decreasing error' (1999, p.4).

The process of testing conclusions is, of course, crucial. Unfortunately, however, there is always some disagreement as to the kinds of things that are to be considered valid criteria for making research judgements. What exactly is an acceptable 'test' that can be applied to your conclusions? So far as scientific research is concerned, the test applied is almost always the degree to which something conforms to a particular theory about causality. Changes take place in phenomena which make sense according to this theory rather than some other one. They are measurable changes, and the fact that they turn out the way that they do demonstrates that the explanation proposed by the theory is the correct one.

Unfortunately, however, the classical scientific approach does not always tell us as much about therapy as it does about other aspects of human reality. This is because not all theories about causality which are mathematically verifiable are adequate explanations of the action of psychotherapy. It is easy enough to demonstrate that psychotherapy changes human behaviour and experience; this can be done by straightforward 'before' and 'after' testing. What is much more difficult is to draw scientific conclusions about how, in fact, it manages to do so.

The main problem confronting research into dramatherapy is that of finding ways of understanding the actual process of healing. As time goes on, this problem becomes more and more pressing. As Gordon Langley says, 'We owe it to our clients to provide them with the best available evidence that our methods are effective, and at the same time if that evidence is less rigorous than it should be, to improve in its accuracy' (1999, p.10). Improving the effectiveness of dramatherapy involves considerably more than simply measuring outcomes, of course. Only by discovering more about the dramatherapy process can we avoid the trap which confronts everybody who wants to 'do research', that of seeking the wrong kind of information about the wrong set of circumstances in the wrong way. Achieving results is not enough, they must be the kind of results which provide real insight into the state of affairs which produced them.

Systematic validation involves the choice of an appropriate research strategy for the task in hand. Grainger (1999a, 1999b) describes several alternative strategies, each of which involves the use of a different 'research orientation':

1   *Quantitative dramatherapy research.* This attempts to draw conclusions about the effectiveness of therapy by measuring its outcome. A cause-and-effect relationship is established along scientific lines, the cause being defined in simple terms as 'the action of the therapy'. This does not need to be investigated, although the experimenter may have some theories about it.

2   *Qualitative dramatherapy research.* This is more concerned with investigating processes involved than establishing degrees of change. It does not depend upon mathematical measurement for the accuracy it claims. The question at issue here is how changes take place, and this can be answered only by the investigator's willingness to surrender scientific objectivity by him or herself 'entering the dramatherapy process'. This does not, however, mean that rules governing the establishment of cause-and-effect linkages have to be abandoned (King, Keohane and Verba 1994).

3    *Practitioner dramatherapy research* is the logical development of (strategy 2), facing the fact that understanding of the reality of human experience is bound to depend primarily on involvement and only secondarily on any 'scientific detachment' the investigator can bring to bear on the situation. We are concerned here with exploring the experience of the whole researcher–researchee situation, rather than trying to stand apart from a particular state of affairs in order to carry out research on it (Robson 1993).

4    *Art-based research* (McNiff 1998). This is the 'approach of preference' for arts therapies research because it holds to the idea that the traditions of enquiry associated with traditional scientific ways of understanding cannot be used to research an artistic medium because they are essentially anti-creativity and pro-systemisation. 'Because of its unwillingness to translate the language of artistic experience into any other kind of code, claiming that the loss of meaning involved in doing this actually destroys the whole purpose of research, art-based research explores experiential transformations without quantifying them' (Grainger 1999b, p.141).

The four approaches tested here are all effective within their own particular spheres of operations – quantitative research for determining measurable changes, qualitative research for investigating the experience of individuals and groups involved in personal and social change, practitioner research for assessing the research situation as a total interpersonal event, art-based research as a way of letting artistic experience speak out for itself. Used selectively, each of these models has something to contribute to the task of finding out what dramatherapy is, what it does and how effectively it does it. Together they form a 'research repertoire' (Grainger 1999b) which a dramatherapist may call upon to tackle problems of formal evaluation, always remembering, of course, that research of any kind involves a lot of hard work and specialised knowledge and should not be undertaken without the support and advice of people who already have some expertise in the field.

For dramatherapists, the art-based approach has some very definite advantages, not only because it treats artistic experience in general as a valid way of making sense of human life, but also because of the kind of artistic experience – drama – that it uses in order to do it. As artistic creativity takes the form of a statement rather than a question or a problem, its particular way of answering questions and solving problems is by demonstrating or presenting rather than arguing. Drama answers questions about life and death by showing us these things in action. It is its nature to do this; we do not have to set about using it in a special way in order to make it work. Dramatherapy is not *applied* drama, but simply the imaginative portrayal of human experience. Making a dramatic model of personal behaviour reveals the questions to be asked and shows the answers *as drama*. Understanding emerges in terms of the dramatic quality of the event; it is the play itself and what happens in it that is assimilated and learned from, and the learning is existential – that is, it is an experience of personal involvement, remembered as an episode in life, not merely an addition to one's store of information. This is why dramatherapy lends itself to art-based research rather than to any other approach: it can only be accurately evaluated by *experiencing the drama* and so taking part in the investigation into being human that it embodies. From this point of view, dramatherapy is that form of art-based research whose medium is drama, and subject matter the world of human relationships that drama presents.

# CHAPTER 10

# Conclusion

The dramatherapy approach is not to do things *to* individuals, but to allow things to happen *between* people. Because it takes the ways in which we present ourselves to one another – and to ourselves – seriously it can be used in all kinds of interpersonal situations where human breakdown has occurred without depriving them of humanness. To regard it as a treatment for specific psychiatric conditions is seriously to limit its usefulness by ignoring its flexibility. Certainly, at first sight, this makes it an obvious treatment of choice for problems involving the ways in which we feel and think about our relationship with the persons and things that constitute our individual worlds. Feelings of hopelessness and inferiority, social anxiety and personal depression, inability to stand up for oneself or the underlying lack of confidence which leads to over-assertion and aggressiveness; inability to make cognitive sense of things that are happening and one's own reactions to them, haunting memories of past failures and crippling fears about the future; an inadequate or almost nonexistent sense of self, of having a personal centre, and a lack of confidence in the value and significance of one's own actions and experiences – all these things, and others like them, are the obvious raw material of dramatherapy.

But the usefulness of dramatherapy is not confined to the medical conditions and types of social breakdown of which these things are the most obvious and important symptoms, and we certainly did not intend to produce a complete map of the territory covered by dramatherapy, which by concentrating on some areas in too much detail, managed at the same time to draw almost equal attention to the things it left out. Our aim, however, is to underline dramatherapy's flexibility not its limitations, although it obviously has some: it cannot totally reverse the effects of psychological trauma, for instance, any more than it can heal physical lesions of any kind. At the same time it can certainly *help* to do a lot of things which appear at first sight to be outside its range of effectiveness. It can set the scene for healing which may require intervention of other kinds – and sometimes setting the scene can be crucial for the success of any actual intervention of a more technical nature. This is true whether we are talking about either psychotherapy or biological medicine. As we have seen, dramatherapy uses imagination to promote realism; it brings home the need for personal healing of all kinds, and at the same time helps us to see ourselves as persons who may contribute to our own healing.

If this appears to confine its effectiveness to situations of physical and/or emotional breakdown, even this is not true – for 'healing' read 'learning'. Dramatherapy helps us to understand. Its healing comes via its ability, at all levels, to teach us about the ways in which our personal worlds meet and interact. Just as it works against any kind of systematic reduction of individuality, so it militates against a solipsistic interpretation of life. Dramatherapy teaches us who – and *where* – we are. Again, it does this by opening the door to discovery of self and other, *setting the scene* for enlightenment. It is for teachers, group leaders, community workers, mediators, social enquirers and facilitators of all kinds (including managers) as well as nurses, doctors and therapists of every description. In fact, for anyone whose purpose, professional or not, is the promotion of person-hood, dramatherapy offers a way of opening up a shared universe – one that is revealed in the actual experience of sharing the very real life of creative imagination.

From this point of view it is a partly theoretical, partly practical, hands-on book, coming as it does directly from the authors' experience of working dramatherapeutically in a whole range of settings and for many different purposes. There are quite a number of books about what dramatherapy itself is – at least, what it sets out to be. We hope that in this book we have drawn attention to the essential flexibility of dramatherapy as a medium of human communication. In describing a number of key aspects of human interpersonal experience – ways in which we normally react to our own and other people's presence in any human situation – we have tried to show how dramatherapy sheds light on that particular area of life. Sometimes the dramatherapy approach to life situations is markedly different from other kinds of interventions. For example, social skills training (discussed in Chapter 2) is a recognised category of task-orientated behaviour modification; dramatherapy, while setting out to enable the same kind of behavioural adjustment, works in its own characteristically dramatherapeutic way. This is true of the relationship between other therapeutic and educational techniques and dramatherapy. Other examples are the meaning-orientated dramatherapy and personal history approaches discussed in Chapters 6 and 7, which deal with the same kinds of subject matter as, respectively, cognitive-behavioural intervention and personal construct therapy. Chapter 4 (on masks) looked at the therapeutic effect of drama in a way that is comparable to, but quite different from, psychodrama. The structures described in this book, although they are concerned with different social and individual situations, are all distinctively dramatherapeutic approaches. As such they are all available for use by anybody who is interested in exploring the ways in which people relate to themselves and one another, whether the underlying purpose of the exercise is to find a way of improving communication within a task-orientated group, or one of identifying the unconscious dynamisms described by psychoanalysis – as in Marina Jenkyns' (1996) object-relations approach to dramatic texts (Chapter 8).

Within the dramatherapy process people come face to face under circumstances that require them to take account of each other's living reality. In such a context we can no longer reduce other people's feelings, ideas and attitudes to other, less subtle and original versions of our own, nor write them off altogether if we can see no way in which they can be made to fit our system. In a dramatherapy workshop the reality of other people and of the things that belong to them must be encountered at first hand. It cannot simply be dismissed, as if life were an exchange of articles in a professional journal. The use of dramatherapy in workshops devised for this kind of exchange of ideas among people with differing attitudes and viewpoints – professional or otherwise – has not been discussed here, although some of the processes described in Chapter 6, in which we looked at individuals and groups occupied in the serious business of discovering meaning in life and death, have an obvious bearing on it. In fact dramatherapy often provides this kind of arena for the exchange of ideas and experiences among people from different professional backgrounds whose ways of looking at things reflect the particular nature of the kinds of work they do and the circumstances in which they do it.

Dramatherapy as a medium for interdisciplinary exchange is starting to draw greater attention as more and more professionals begin to discover that what they once dismissed as a 'fringe' therapy, likely to be useful only in a very limited number of cases and under special circumstances (usually when respectable scientific procedures had been tried out and found unsuccessful), is able to open doors which have long been firmly shut to them simply because it can give a valuable new dimension to their normal ways of working – a flexibility and spontaneity which, by humanising the way in which it is delivered, can greatly extend its scope.

This does not mean, of course, that dramatherapy should be used thoughtlessly or automatically applied in every situation involving a group of people where there might be some difficulty in 'getting things off the ground'. Dramatherapy has its own integrity, in the sense of being a process rather than a technique. As we saw in Chapter 2, a dramatherapy session is a free-standing event, with a beginning, a middle and an end. For an interpersonal event to be dramatherapeutic it must reproduce this sense of movement into and out of a time of concentrated awareness of one's own and other people's immediate experience, however uncomfortable and disturbing this should turn out to be. It is quite possible and certainly not unusual for people to include some features of dramatherapy sessions in the plans they are making for meetings not intended to be even implicitly therapeutic – and to discover that the thoughts and feelings expressed by those present are dramatically changed in the direction of increased frankness and self-disclosure. At the same time, some of the things that have come to be regarded as typical ingredients of drama-therapy – group games, role-reversal exercises, mirroring, speaking as if you were your neighbour in order to express what you sense he or she is feeling but cannot put into words ('ego-ing'), leaving a chair empty in order to be able to address an invisible person imagined to be sitting there – are by no means original to dramatherapy and are certainly not confined to it. These techniques and others like them are carefully devised ways of working towards the central purpose, which is the imaginative liberation of personhood. They are included in dramatherapy because they are useful to this end but are certainly not essential to it and should not be allowed to obscure the overall process of *change through imaginative experience* mediated by the symbolic shape of the whole session. It can only be hoped that people interested enough to include specific dramatherapy techniques in their current practice with the limited intention of making what they are already doing work better will be encouraged to look more deeply into what it is they are using and so discover its ability to transform an entire approach, rather than simply adding to the effectiveness of the ways in which it already functions. All the same, there is no doubt that these individual techniques are useful in themselves – which is how they found their way into dramatherapy in the first place.

Certainly the dramatherapy model has been found extremely useful by members of other professions – psychologists, teachers, community workers, psychiatric nurses and occupational therapists are just a few of the representatives of other disciplines in which individual practitioners have become so involved in this approach that they have undertaken special training and can now call themselves genuine inter-professionals and not just tourists. To be a dramatherapy tourist, however, can be a refreshing and deeply stimulating experience, just so long as you are willing to take in the landscape itself and not simply its most obvious landmarks. What we have tried to get across in this book is the expansive spirit of dramatherapy; its fundamental flexibility rather than its availability as a collection of techniques, a kind of therapeutic tool-box. This flexibility comes from the fact that it is based on a fundamental human principle – the way in which we use imagination to transform and humanise the world we live in. This is the way people learn to heal themselves; the way that they *learn to be people* in powerful contrast to the private fantasy solutions we use to avoid contact with reality in our efforts to hide from life. This is the public use of creative imagination, to join not to divide, bringing us into healing contact with one another and with ourselves. In dramatherapy we find ways of contacting life, getting a grip on realities that need to be seen as a whole, as part of being human. The structure of dramatherapy presents life within a context of meaning and purpose – things which for human beings are intrinsically bound up with and dependent on *imagination*.

This book, then, is an attempt to present dramatherapy as it is – a structure for imaginative healing. As such it is as flexible as our imagination will let it be. This does not mean that it is vague or airy-fairy in any way. Because it is organised as a way in which people are enabled to communicate with one another, its effectiveness depends on the clarity with which it presents its messages about the things involved in being human. These messages may not always be spelt out in so many words; but the use of words can itself be very misleading and people have a tendency to make their own kind of sense out of things other people say to them – particularly when what is said concerns their most sensitive thoughts and feelings regarding themselves and their personal worlds. In dramatherapy we are not limited by our ability to express ourselves clearly and accurately on subjects we have been taught to regard as beyond the range of the medically or psychologically uninitiated; nor do we have to suffer the indignity of being clinically 'understood' without having been given a realistic opportunity to show who we are and how it is with us. The structure of dramatherapy is designed to encourage us to create the kind of shared space we need in order to present ourselves in situations involving other people in which we may be able to reveal the living truth about us – the quality of our present and past experience – rather than relying on descriptions of ourselves, either other people's or our own, whose main virtue often seems to be the ease with which they fit into ready-made categories used to explain human behaviour.

On the other hand, dramatherapy does not rule out the necessity to think logically and clearly (or as logically and clearly as we can manage to think) about things that concern us, and particularly the things that have revealed themselves to us in the course of our exploration into what it feels like to share in the drama of being together. Here again, the shape of a dramatherapy session provides us with an opportunity to look back on an experience we have recently been through together with a degree of calmness and objectivity which we cannot manage when we are up to our necks in things, stuck right in the middle of the action. The safe space designed to give us the confidence we need to become involved can also encourage us to sit back and reflect on what being involved actually felt like, and how we and the other people present reacted to the situation. The concluding part of a dramatherapy experience can be a favourable time for drawing conclusions, not only about the session but also about life itself and our most sensitive feelings about being human: life from the inside, in fact. People engaged in carrying out research into dramatherapy con-centrate on this part because of the frankness and spontaneity of the testimony provided by those who have been personally involved in whatever has been going on in the main body of the session. These are the ideas and feelings that we carry away with us from the experience; these and a gallery of images, some of which flit across our mental screen so rapidly that we are unable to pin them down, some we manage to keep hold of so that we can enjoy looking at them again whenever we want to, some which stay in our minds at an unconscious level, affecting our attitude to life in ways that are not measurable.

All this is part of the process of readjustment to what we usually call the 'real' world outside the charmed circle of imaginative participation, although 'ordinary' would be better than 'real'. Our ability to 'co-imagine' with other people so that we actually create a shared scenario introduces us to a way of knowing in which we experience life by participating in it, rather than just thinking about it. These experiences must be consolidated and established as part of our own individual history, our sense of being people who have done certain things and to whom certain things have happened. The poet Wordsworth defined poetry as 'emotion recollected in tranquillity' (1800, p.171). To co-imagine in this way, and then to take time quietly mulling over where we have been and who we have met there, is to produce the raw material of poetry.

As we said at the beginning of this book, dramatherapy hangs together as a complete happening, with a beginning, a middle and an end. To divide it up is to take away its impact and reduce its power to heal. The world of imagination which comes into being as a result of the decision to imagine together is something which must be consciously and deliberately entered upon, and just and consciously and deliberately left behind afterwards. More time may be spent in working together than in preparing to do so and establishing an ending; but the processes of starting and stopping define the nature of what happens between, giving it an identity and a value as something deliberately undertaken, something important carried out by the people present. This is particularly important, because imagination sees no reason to restrict its operations unless it is deliberately associated with specific occasions. It cannot be tied down, but it can be bracketed off, focused (which is why we are able to enjoy works of art).

On the other hand it is also vitally important for the group leader to allow the conversation in this part of the session to move wherever it seems to want to go. Certainly leaders may feel some need to reassure themselves by asking 'How did it go?', hoping it went well, and they will say so. This, however, is not the main point of the exercise. The purpose of drama-therapy is not necessarily to provide people with 'a good trip'. Some of the country you have been travelling through together will have been hard going, at least for some of those taking part. You would not have gone there unless you felt safe. All the same, you have been coming into contact with things about yourself and other people which may have been painful and challenging. Now you have come out on the other side. Some at least of the people in the group may feel that they have not emerged completely unscathed. Now is the time to lick your wounds. It has been specifically provided for this purpose; the leader's nervousness or fear of having to listen to what may seem to be a criticism should not be allowed to get in the way. This is not ordinary criticism, in any case. It is more likely to be a straightforward reaction on the part of people who feel that they may have shown more of themselves than they feel entirely comfortable about – much more, in fact, than they are used to showing, either to other people or to themselves!

People need time to adjust to what you have all co-operated in making into an emotional experience of some power. In the final part of the session, time is provided along with the permission to do this publicly by sharing one's feelings with the group. This is no time, however, for the group leader to take offence because people are not happy with the way they feel just at present. The group is still there; it has not broken up yet. People are still supporting one another simply by being together in the group. In fact, they are more help to one another than they were able to be at the beginning. They can say things about themselves and the way they feel which were beyond them then – and they can say them differently now. This is all part of the session itself. In this way the shape of dramatherapy enables sensitive people to adjust to going out into the world again.

Not that this is ever easy, even for those who have had an easier passage through the session. It is a well-known characteristic of working in groups that the more one enjoys the session the harder it is to let go of it and say goodbye. (Writing this book has been a lot like that, too.) This seems to be true of every experience of sharing with other people in which the relationship has grown and developed over time. A dramatherapy session may last only hour or two, but its structure is designed to embody a participant's hope of personal transformation by taking him or her on a journey into and out of a focused emotional experience so as to exert pressure on current ways of feeling, thinking and, consequently, behaving.

To some extent everyone involved has come into contact with what Nigel Tubbs calls 'the roaring and roasting of the broken middle' (1998, p.34). What has made the experience tolerable has been the sense of 'all being in it together'; now they have to say goodbye to each other and go their separate ways, and the sense of being on one's own is greatly magnified. Loneliness and a sense of frailty go hand in hand, of course. As Foulkes and Anthony put it, 'Endings seem to lead to the futility of life and the inevitability of death' (1957, p.168).

Foulkes and Anthony (1957) were writing about group psychotherapy. One of the things they stress, as does Irvin Yalom (1985) writing some years later, is the sheer emotional support given by the fact of being in a group, even if it only consists of three or four people. When dramatherapy is done with a single client this openness to the presence of others has to be created in the imagination of client and therapist; but it is always there and always essential to the process of healing. These are people who are here in the present moment, here with us now, whether or not they possess flesh and blood bodies; as we have seen, a lot of very powerful work can be done with dolls and puppets. They may recall incidents and relationships that belong to the past; but the process of dramatherapy makes that belonging a matter of what is actually taking place here, in the dramatherapy space, wherever that may be. Dramatherapy is a present happening in a special sense, one that distinguishes it from other kinds of therapy taking place in groups. Analytic group therapy in particular aims at transferring (in the Freudian sense) significant relationships which developed in the past lives of those taking part into the present situation within the group. The fact that it is a group is regarded as crucial because it lifts the load of transferred feeling from the shoulders of the therapist and distributes it among the group members, so that they all take on roles from the past, each of them becoming unconsciously involved in a network of personal relationships whose meaning is drawn from their individual histories, to be lived over again in the specially protected – and protective – circumstances of the group.

The difference with regard to dramatherapy lies in the basic nature of drama – that it is something done, acted out. It does not simply allow past things to be present, it actually *presents* them as if they are happening now. The foundation of some of the ideas people have about the kind of role they choose to take on, or emotion or idea they set about expressing in dramatic form in a dramatherapy session, may well be transferential in this psychoanalytic sense – given the nature of human family relationships it would be hard to imagine how it could avoid being – and this may be pointed out in the part of the session when things like this are looked at and pondered on. The source of dramatherapy's power to heal is not located here, however, but in the dramatic action itself, the realisation of relationship in imaginative settings consciously created for the purpose by the people taking part. Writers on the subject of group therapy from Bion (1961) onwards have seen much more in the experience than simply an opportunity to analyse the psychic processes of individual group members. For Yalom, the heart of group healing lies in 'the affective sharing of one's inner world' (1985, p.50). Dramatherapy maximises the possibility of sharing by making use of one of the most powerful and more essentially human ways of communicating the reality of our personal experience: drama and theatre. Things are not simply remembered, but remembered and relived. The process of co-imagination and co-creation allows us to draw nearer to the things we are beginning to re-remember than any amount of talking about them can do; the ability to embody our free associations within a living context of other people gives them an immediacy and vividness, a sense of personal significance that belongs only to drama, the medium in which we *do* the meaning of things, rather than just thinking about it and trying to describe it.

This, of course, is the motivation behind Moreno's invention of psychodrama (Fox 1987). The kinds of approaches described in this book are not intended to make use of drama in the direct and intensive way that psychodrama does. They do not focus on the circumstances of an individual's personal experience, harnessing the imaginative potential of everybody present for the purpose of creating a living autobiography of the protagonist. Dramatherapy is neither so direct nor so intensive as that. The dramas and scenarios it works with emerge from the imaginative life of those present, just as they do in classical psychodrama; but their subject matter is unlikely to be conceived as an individual's personal story and, in fact, many of the people whom dramatherapy aims at reaching and helping would be greatly alarmed by such an idea, and probably refuse to take part. Dramatherapy's scenarios emerge from shared experience. They represent an understanding of or an insight into the business of living and dying which can be expressed in terms of dramatic interaction on behalf of everyone present. They are not *about* anyone present, however. Rather, they are about individual experiences and meanings held in common. Because of this, they may be personally appropriated by any or all of the people present as particular expressions of their own experience. The act of appropriation, of imaginative identification with some other person or situation 'in' the drama, is carried out by the individuals themselves. It is based on recognition and insight, and calls directly on our imagination and empathy, all of which emerge during the course of the session rather than being engineered into it in accordance with some set of original specifications. Sometimes the effect can be as powerful as psychodrama; sometimes – quite often – it is less striking. It is always free, however. It is also more authentically theatrical. After all, we do not visit theatres to see plays based explicitly upon ourselves; the effect on our state of mind would certainly be devastating if we did! Psychodrama clients are shielded from this kind of public exposure, certainly, but the emotional impact of the psychodramatic experience can be overwhelming for very vulnerable people. Allowing yourself to get involved in things that are happening to somebody whom you perceive as 'like me but not me' is much less threatening and may be equally effective.

'Like me but not me.' As we have been saying all along, the underlying principle of any kind of dramatherapy is imaginative involvement in interpersonal process. Dramatherapy works because it is dramatic. However restrained, limited or low-key a dramatherapy process may be, it always involves a relationship between people that is experienced in the unique way that drama is always experienced; that is, as imaginative involvement in interpersonal situations which are not explicitly our business, *but which we make our business through becoming personally involved in them*. In other words, drama depends on the ability to identify with other people. This basic fact may be described in a number of ways, some of which may permit it to be explained according to a particular psychological model – as, for instance, social learning, reinforced behavioural response (in which the imagined scenario provides the conditioned stimulus), psychological modelling or a distributed form of psychodynamic transference. In the light of the actual experience of dramatherapy, however, none of these explanations quite fit the bill. This is because all of them tend to regard dramatic structure as a way of providing opportunities for learning new patterns of behaviour which could be and usually are learned in other ways and under other circumstances. For them, drama is simply a convenient tool for learning by conscious association, or unconscious identification, or the straightforward contiguity of operant and reward.

Dramatherapists, however, know that what happens in drama is more than this. The conscious action of identification which identifies genuine dramatic experience is neither intentional nor automatic. The drama invites this kind of understanding but in no way imposes it. The learning that takes place – or does not take place – in drama is learning by discovery. We discover that a situation speaks to us or that a person reminds us of someone we know. It is not so much a matter of the assimilation of a new learning – although that certainly happens – as the recognition of old understanding. We see ourselves in the play because we choose to do so, for no other reason. It may not even be anybody remotely resembling us, confronted by a set of circumstances we have never faced, and could never imagine ourselves facing; never, that is, until now. The reason why drama 'heals our emotions', as Aristotle puts it, is because it leaves us free to respond to others – and ourselves seen from another viewpoint, understood in another context – without imposing its meanings on us along with the behaviour required by them. From this point of view, it could be said that drama has as much to do with love as with rationality, at least in the way it functions. Then again, however skilfully and thoughtfully it is presented, it remains art rather than science.

In dramatherapy, the skill lies in managing to achieve the psychological equilibrium of safety and danger – the abandonment of defensiveness that allows a cathartic release of feeling lies in drama itself. Here, the feeling is one of empathetic involvement, and the way it is released is by means of the imaginative 'frame' of drama, the distance that encourages relationship. The relationship may be with other people or with psychologically alienated parts of oneself. Foulkes and Anthony (1957), writing about group analysis, describe how 'in the permissiveness and secure atmosphere of the group [an individual] may let down the iron curtain of repression and expose his vulnerability' (1957, p.202). Whether or not we wish to talk in terms of repression, the fact remains that the presence of other people can make us feel vulnerable and defensive, causing us to withdraw from the kind of contact with other people, the kind of human *reality*, which our humanness needs in order to grow and flourish – in order to recover. This is abundantly true in every situation that involves psycho-therapy. Before real healing can take place something must be there to encourage our responsiveness. Nowhere does this happen more strikingly – and consistently – than in dramatherapy.

# References

Andersen-Warren, M. (1991) *'The Revenger's Tragedy:* From spectators to participants.' *Dramatherapy 14,* 2, 4–8.

Andersen-Warren, M. (1996) 'Therapeutic theatre.' In S. Mitchell (ed) *Dramatherapy: Clinical Studies.* London: Jessica Kingsley Publishers.

Beckett, S. (1986) 'Waiting for Godot.' In *The Complete Dramatic Works.* London: Faber.

Berger, P. (1967) *The Social Reality of Religion.* Harmondsworth: Penguin.

Bion, W.R. (1961) *Experiences in Groups.* London: Tavistock.

Blatner, A. (1997) *Acting-In.* London: Free Association Books.

Blatner, A. and Blatner, A. (1988) *The Art of Play.* New York: Human Sciences.

Boal, A. (1979) *Theatre of the Oppressed.* London: Pluto.

Boal, A. (1992) *Games for Actors and Non-Actors.* London: Routledge.

Boal, A. (1995) *The Rainbow of Desire.* London: Routledge.

Brecht, B. (1964) *Brecht on Theatre.* New York: Hill and Wang.

Brook, E.N. (1979) *Horrid Laughter in Jacobean Tragedy.* London: Open Books.

Brook, P. (1968) *The Empty Space.* London: MacGibbon & Kee.

Buber, M. (1957) *Pointing the Way.* London: Routledge.

Butcher, S.H. (1951) *A Commentary on Aristotle's Poetics.* New York: Dover.

Carroll, L. (1980) *The Hunting of the Snark.* London: W.H.Smith/Windward. (Originally published in 1876.)

Cattanach, A. (1992) *Play Therapy with Abused Children.* London: Jessica Kingsley Publishers.

Coleridge, S.T. (1991) *Biographia Literaria* (ed. G. Watson). London: Dent. (Originally published in 1817.)

Cox, M. (1978) *Coding the Therapeutic Process.* London: Routledge.

Cox, M. and Theilgaard, A. (1987) *Mutative Metaphors in Psychotherapy.* London: Tavistock.

Crites, S. (1986) 'Storytime: Recollecting the past and projecting the future.' In T.R. Sarbin (ed) *Narrative Psychology.* New York: Praeger.

Duggan, M. and Grainger, R. (1997) *Imagination, Identification and Catharsis in Theatre and Therapy.* London: Jessica Kingsley Publishers.

Elam, K. (1988) *Semiotics of Theatre and Drama.* London: Routledge.

Eliade, M. (1958) *Patterns in Comparative Religion.* London: Sheed & Ward.

Eliade, M. (1968) *Myths, Dreams and Mysteries.* London: Collins.

Eliot, T.S. (1955) *Murder in the Cathedral.* London: Faber.

Erikson, E. (1965) *Childhood and Society.* Harmondsworth: Penguin.

Fernstein, D. and Krippner, S. (1989) *Personal Mythology.* London: Unwin.

Flowers, J.V. (1975) 'Stimulation and role playing methods.' In F.H. Kanfer and A.P. Goldstein (eds) *Helping People Change.* Oxford: Pergamon.

Foulkes, S.H. and Anthony, E.J. (1957) *Group Psychotherapy.* Harmondsworth: Penguin.

Fox, J. (ed) (1987) *The Esssential Moreno.* New York: Springer.

Frankl, V. (1964) *Man's Search for Meaning.* London: Hodder.

Freud, S. (1895) 'On the grounds for detaching a particular syndrome from neurasthenia under the description "Anxiety Neurosis".' In *Standard Edition*, vol. 3. London: Hogarth Press.

Freud, S. (1909) 'Some general remarks on hysterical attacks.' In *Standard Edition*, vol. 9. London: Hogarth Press.

Gardiner, V. (1987) 'Building out of "Blocks".' *Dramatherapy 10*, 2, 8–16.

Gersie, A. and King, N. (1990) *Storymaking in Education and Therapy.* London: Jessica Kingsley Publishers.

Gibbon, B. (ed) (1967) *The Revenger's Tragedy.* London: New Mermaid Books.

Goffman, E. (1986) *Frame Analysis.* Boston, MA: Northeastern University Press.

Goffman, E. (1990) *The Presentation of Self in Everyday Life.* Harmondsworth: Penguin.

Grainger, R. (1990) *Drama and Healing.* London: Jessica Kingsley Publishers.

Grainger, R. (1995) *The Glass of Heaven.* London: Jessica Kingsley Publishers.

Grainger, R. (1999a) 'Supervision and consultancy of art-based research.' In E. Tselikas-Portmann (ed) *Supervision and Dramatherapy.* London: Jessica Kingsley Publishers.

Grainger, R. (1999b) *Researching the Arts Therapies: A Dramatherapist's Perspective.* London: Jessica Kingsley Publishers.

Graves, R. (1981) *Greek Myths.* London: Cassell.

Jacobi, J. (1976) *Masks of the Soul.* London: Darton, Longman & Todd.

Jenkyns, M. (1996) *The Play's the Thing.* London: Routledge.

Jennings, S. (1986) *Creative Drama in Groupwork.* London: Winslow.

Jennings, S. (1990) *Dramatherapy with Families, Groups and Individuals: Waiting in the Wings.* London: Jessica Kingsley Publishers.

Johnstone, K. (1981) *Impro: Improvisation and the Theatre.* London: Methuen.

Jones, P. (1995) *Drama as Therapy: Theatre as Living.* London: Routledge.

Jourard, S.M. (1964) *The Transparent Self.* New York: Norton.

Kelly, G.A. (1955) *The Psychology of Personal Constructs.* New York: Norton.

Kelly, G.A. (1963) *A Theory of Personality.* New York: Norton.

King, L., Keohane, K.O. and Verba, S. (1994) *Designing Social Enquiry.* Princeton, NJ: Princeton University Press.

Klein, M. (1988) *Love, Guild and Reparation.* London: Virago.

Landy, R.J. (1993) *Persona and Performance.* London: Jessica Kingsley Publishers.

Langley, D. (1983) *Dramatherapy and Psychiatry.* London: Croom Helm.

Langley, G. (1999) 'Research methods and models: Must methods match the model?' *European Consortium for Arts Therapies*, Munster.

Lewis, G. (1980) *The Day of Shining Red.* Cambridge: Cambridge University Press.

Lucas, F.L. (1946) *Tragedy.* London: Hogarth Press.

Mackewn, J. (1997) *Developing Gestalt Counselling.* London: Sage.

Mair, M. (1989) *Between Psychology and Psychotherapy.* London: Routledge.

McNiff, S. (1998) *Art-Based Research.* London: Jessica Kingsley Publishers.

May, R. (1975) *The Courage to Create.* London: Collins.

Moreno, J. (1977) *Psychodrama,* vol. 1. New York: Beacon House.

Murray, H.A. (ed) (1960) *Myth and Mythmaking.* New York: Braziller.

Nilsson, M.P. (1964) *A History of Greek Religion.* New York: Norton.

Nygaard, J. (1994) 'The Theatre as a Seismograph of Society.' Paper delivered at the twelfth World Congress of the International Federation for Theatre Research. Moscow 1994.

Perls, F. (1948) 'Theory and technique of personal integration.' *American Journal of Psychotherapy 2,* 565–586.

Phelps, S. and Austin, A. (1988) *The Assertive Woman.* London: Arlington.

Robson, C. (1993) *Real World Research.* Oxford: Blackwell.

Rowan, J. (1993) *The Transpersonal.* London: Routledge.

Sarason, S. (1990) *The Challenge of Art to Psychology.* New Haven: Yale University Press.

Saroyan, W. (1996) *The Time of Your Life: A Comedy.* London: French.

Scheff, T.J. (1979) *Catharsis in Healing, Ritual and Drama.* Berkeley, CA: University of California Press.

Searles, H. (1965) 'The informational value of the supervisor's emotional experience.' In H. Searles (ed) *Collected Papers on Schizophrenia and Related Subjects.* London: Hogarth Press.

Shohet, R. and Hawkins, P. (1989) *Supervision in the Helping Professions.* Milton Keynes: Open University Press.

Slade, P. (1995) *Child Play.* London: Jessica Kingsley Publishers.

Sorrell, W. (1973) *The Other Face: The Mask in the Arts.* London: Thames & Hudson.

Stanislavksi, C. (1948) *An Actor Prepares* (trans. E.R. Hapgood). New York: Theatre Arts Books.

Thorne, B. (1997) 'Spiritual responsibility in a secular profession.' In I. Horton and V. Varma (eds) *The Needs of Counsellors and Psychotherapists.* London: Sage.

Tillich, P. (1958) *The Dynamics of Faith.* New York: Harper & Row.

Tubbs, N. (1998) 'What Is Love's Work?' *Women: A Cultural Review 19,* 1, 34–36.

Turner, V. (1974) *The Ritual Process.* Harmondsworth: Penguin.

Van Gennep, A. (1960) *The Rites of Passage* (trans. M.B. Vizedom and G.L. Caffee). London: Routledge.

Wickham, G. (1959) *Early English Stages 1300–1600.* London: Methuen.

Wilshire, M. (1982) *Role Playing and Identity.* Bloomington, IN: University of Indiana Press.

Winnicott, D.W. (1960) 'Ego distortion in terms of true and false self.' In *The Maturational Processes and the Facilitating Environment* (1958). London: Hogarth Press.

Winnicott, D.W. (1971) *Playing and Reality.* London: Tavistock.

Wordsworth, W. (1800) 'Preface to Lyrical Ballads.' In N. Smith (1921) *Wordsworth.* Oxford: Oxford University Press.

Yalom, I. (1985) *The Theory and Practice of Group Psychotherapy.* New York: Basic Books.

# Subject Index

# Author Index